Medicines, Patients, and the Gaps Between

Nadir Kheir

Medicines, Patients, and the Gaps Between

A Researcher's Reflections on What We Found, What We Missed, and What Remains

Springer

Nadir Kheir
School of Pharmacy and Biomedical
Sciences
Division of Health University of Waikato
Hamilton, Waikato, New Zealand

Ajman University
Ajman, UAE

ISBN 978-981-92-5394-4 ISBN 978-981-92-5395-1 (eBook)
https://doi.org/10.1007/978-981-92-5395-1

This Springer imprint is published by the registered company Springer Nature Singapore Pte Ltd.
The registered company address is: 152 Beach Road, #21-01/04 Gateway East, Singapore 189721, Singapore

To my students, colleagues and mentors, who shaped this work as much as I did, and from whom I am still learning. I am grateful to my family, who lived through the years this work took without ever asking to be part of it. And, most of all, to the patients, whose experiences are the reason this research existed in the first place; every finding in this book began with them, whether or not they ever knew it.

Preface: An Unusual Kind of Accounting

Research papers are written to report what was found. This book is written to reckon with what that means, looking back across more than two decades of pharmacy practice research conducted in Qatar, the United Arab Emirates, New Zealand and beyond, and asking a set of questions that the papers themselves could not ask: What did we actually achieve? What did we miss and why? What did the field learn and what has it stubbornly refused to learn? What remains urgently unfinished?

This book occupies a genre that barely exists in the health sciences, though I believe it should: the research retrospective, written from the inside by someone who conducted the work and can therefore speak about it with an honesty that external reviewers, however rigorous, cannot quite reach. I have been a pharmacist, an educator and a researcher. I have contributed in designing studies, written protocols, supervised graduate students and watched, sometimes with satisfaction and sometimes with genuine frustration, as findings that seemed important to us quietly disappeared into the literature without changing much of anything. This book is my attempt to make sense of all of that, not as personal history, but as a contribution to how the pharmacy research community thinks about its own work and its own responsibilities.

Each chapter of this book is built around a specific published study or cluster of studies to which the author contributed. The anchor publication is named, cited in full, and its findings stated accurately. What follows is not a summary of that paper, but the story behind it: the institutional context in which it was conceived, the methodological choices it made, the constraints it worked within and the questions it could not answer. Then comes the critical reckoning: what did the study miss, and what did the gap between its findings and clinical practice cost? And finally, each chapter traces where the publication travelled in the scholarly literature after it appeared, noting the research it entered, the debates it touched and, where the record permits, the directions in which subsequent work moved. This is not a claim to know why any given researcher cited any given paper. Citations are often opportunistic, contextual or simply the best available reference in a particular vicinity. What the citation record does allow is a partial picture of the field's movement, a way of asking whether the problems the original research identified were subsequently engaged with, confirmed, challenged or quietly set aside. What complicates this picture further is that pharmacy and health services research has never developed a validated measure of the impact a piece of research has made on practice; in the absence of such a measure, the citation record, imperfect as it is, remains the most tractable proxy available, a limitation this book returns to directly in its closing chapter.

This full-circle architecture, from anchor publication through the story behind it, through honest reflection on its limits, through the field's response, to what remains undone, is the book's core structural contribution. It is what distinguishes it from a memoir, which offers narrative without evidence; from a systematic review, which offers evidence without voice; and from a textbook, which offers guidance without accountability. What it offers instead is a researcher holding his own work to account.

A note on authorship and reflexivity: The research described in this book was, in most cases, collaborative. I worked with gifted co-investigators, supervisors, students and colleagues across several countries, and their contributions were real and indispensable. Where I speak in the first person, I am speaking about my own role, my own perspective and my own reflections. I am not claiming sole credit for the work, nor am I speaking on behalf of collaborators who might, entirely reasonably, reflect on the same studies in different ways. The retrospective judgements here are mine.

A note on the concentration of this book's evidence base: A reader familiar with the author's career will notice that the majority of publications discussed in these pages originate from the decade spent at the College of Pharmacy at Qatar University. This concentration is not accidental, and Chap. 6 explains the institutional conditions that made it so productive.

A note on the citation trail: Each chapter draws on searches of Google Scholar, PubMed and Semantic Scholar to trace where the anchor publications appeared in subsequent scholarship. These trails are reported honestly: where a paper was included in a systematic review, or cited in a follow-up trial, or carried into a different country or clinical context, that is noted and its significance reflected upon. Where citations are thin, or where the subsequent literature confirmed the problem without resolving it, that too is acknowledged. The citation record is not treated here as proof that the research mattered. It is treated as one imperfect lens, through which the field's engagement with a problem can be observed.

A note on geographical scope: This book draws primarily on research conducted in the Arab Middle East, particularly in Qatar, and on related work in New Zealand and the UAE. The Middle East has been substantially understudied in the pharmacy and health services research literature, relative to its epidemiological significance, its rapidly evolving health systems and the genuine complexity of practising pharmacy in multicultural, multilingual, resource-variable environments.

Throughout this book, publications authored or co-authored by the author are marked with an asterisk (*) in each chapter's reference list. This convention is applied consistently across all 12 chapters.

Hamilton, Waikato, New Zealand Nadir Kheir

Introduction: The Gap That Would Not Close

A Different Kind of Book

Academic publishing has well-established genres, each with its own conventions, its own audience expectations and its own relationship to evidence. The typical textbook organises established knowledge for the learner. The systematic review synthesises existing findings for the practitioner and researcher. The memoir narrates a professional life for the general reader. The collected works assembles an author's publications for archival and retrospective purposes. Each of these forms has genuine value. None of them asks the question this book asks.

This book belongs to a genre that barely exists in the health sciences, though I believe it should: the research retrospective. It is not a memoir, because it is organised around published evidence rather than personal narrative, and because its primary obligation is to the scholarly record rather than to the author's experience of living. It is not a systematic review, because it does not pretend to objectivity or to the elimination of the author's perspective; on the contrary, the author's perspective is the point. It is not a collection of works, because it does not simply reproduce or summarise what was published; it subjects those publications to the kind of critical interrogation that the publications themselves, for reasons of genre and brevity, could not provide. And it is not a textbook, because it does not offer established knowledge with the confidence of settled understanding. It offers, instead, something considerably more uncomfortable: a senior researcher's honest accounting of what a substantial body of work actually achieved, where it fell short and what it has left unfinished. In that sense, it is a disruptive scholarly genre that challenges conventional reflexivity in health sciences scholarship by turning the critical lens inward, onto the researcher's own body of work.

Of the four distinctions drawn above, the one from memoir is the one most easily missed, precisely because this book is written in the first person and draws on lived professional experience, the very material memoir is built from.

What separates it is method, not disclaimer: every claim here is anchored to a named, dated, peer-reviewed publication and traced afterward through its citation record rather than through recollection. A memoir is free to say what a study meant to its author. This book instead asks what became of the problem the study identified in the published record that followed it, a question memoir has neither the mechanism nor the obligation to ask. The first-person voice supplies context for the evidence; it does not stand in for it.

The Connecting Thread

The 12 chapters of this book address topics that appear, at first glance, to be diverse: pharmaceutical care philosophy in the Middle East, medication-related burden, quality of life measurement, pharmacist-delivered clinical interventions, counselling practice in community pharmacies, pharmacy education, research capacity building, medication adherence, caregiver wellbeing, tobacco control and medicines access during COVID-19. A reviewer encountering this list might reasonably ask what connects them. The answer is a single, persistent, structurally embedded problem that each research programme approached from a different angle, named with different precision, and ultimately failed, as each study must, to fully resolve.

The idea for this book did not begin with an observation about the pharmacy profession. It began with a more uncomfortable recognition: that across more than two decades of research, we had identified problems, generated findings, made recommendations and moved on, without ever systematically returning to ask whether any of it had changed anything. This book does not claim to have closed that gap. What it attempts is the prior and necessary step: returning to the publications, reading them honestly against what followed and making the incompleteness visible. That, in itself, is rarer in the health sciences than it should be, and it is a more honest account of what a research retrospective requires than any claim about the profession's shortcomings could provide.

Across the 12 chapters that follow, that gap reveals itself in three distinct but related themes, each encountered independently in different research programmes, across different countries and patient populations, yet each pointing towards the same structural failure. The first theme is the evidence–practice gap: the distance between what the research shows is achievable and what practitioners consistently deliver in everyday clinical encounters. Chapter 5 documents this with precision in the simulated patient study of counselling practice in Qatar: pharmacists who were trained to provide pharmaceutical care, who worked in a system that aspired to pharmaceutical care as its professional standard, and who nonetheless failed to demonstrate adequate inhaler technique to 93.8% of patients presenting with asthma. Chapter 8 documents it through the adherence barrier studies: patients who understood they needed to take their medications, who were attending healthcare clinics regularly and who were nonetheless non-adherent at rates that the healthcare system had not systematically acted to address. Chapter 10 documents it in tobacco control: warnings that increased cessation intentions among smokers who read them, in the absence of the cessation support infrastructure that would have allowed those intentions to become behaviour.

The second theme is the education–environment gap: the distance between the professional formation that pharmacy graduates receive and the practice environment that awaits them. Chapter 1 documents the structural decoupling of education and practice across the Arabic-speaking Middle East over two decades of attempted pharmaceutical care reform. Chapter 6 documents it within a single institution: graduates of a programme that had received the highest international accreditations, who were among the best-prepared pharmacy graduates in the region, and who chose, almost unanimously, not to enter the community pharmacy setting where patient need was the greatest, because the structural conditions of that setting contradicted everything their education had taught them to value. Chapter 7 documents its consequences for research capacity: pharmacists who could be trained to think like scientists, but who returned to practice environments that offered no protected time, no research infrastructure and no professional expectation that scientific inquiry was part of their role.

The third theme is the measurement–action gap: the distance between documenting a problem with precision and building the evidence that something can be done about it. Chapter 2 documents the medication-related burden of patients with non-communicable diseases in Qatar's primary care system, with validated instruments in Arabic and statistically significant associations with adherence, but without the intervention studies that would establish whether pharmacist-led burden assessment and management could change clinical outcomes. Chapter 3 documents improvements in asthma quality of life through pharmaceutical care in New Zealand, while acknowledging that the service demonstrated in a rigorous demonstration project did not become embedded in routine practice. Chapter 9 documents the quality of life burden on caregivers of children with autism, providing a baseline that has not been followed by the intervention evidence that would address what was measured.

These three themes are not independent. They are manifestations of the same structural failure: a profession that has developed, across more than three decades of pharmaceutical care reform, a sophisticated understanding of what it should do for patients, without yet constructing the regulatory, financial, organisational and educational infrastructure that would allow it to do so consistently, at scale, in the practice settings where the need is greatest. That is the argument that runs through this book, and it is an argument that emerges not from a single perspective or a single country but from a research programme conducted across countries, practice settings and patient populations.

Selecting Publications

The publications examined in this book were selected on three criteria. First, they represent the anchor publications of the author's substantive research programmes: not every paper written during a career, but the studies that defined research directions, generated the most significant findings and attracted the most sustained engagement from the field. Second, they span the full breadth of the research programme, from outcome measurement methodology to clinical intervention evaluation to pharmacy education research to public health synthesis, so that the retrospective account is genuinely representative of the scholarly contribution rather than a selective highlight reel. Third, they lend themselves to the full-circle analysis that this book's structure requires: they can be examined not only for what they found but also for what the field subsequently did with those findings, and for what they left unresolved.

The decision to write this book now, at this particular point in a research career, reflects a conviction that has grown over many years of reading the pharmacy practice literature: that the field's *publish-and-move-on* culture is among the most significant obstacles to the cumulative knowledge that genuine professional improvement requires. A research programme that produces publications without examining what those publications achieved, whether the problems they identified have been addressed or whether the same findings are being rediscovered, at cost, by subsequent researchers who did not know they existed, is not building knowledge in any durable sense. It is accumulating a literature. Building knowledge requires exactly what this book attempts: looking back at what was done, asking what it actually accomplished, naming what was missed and identifying what remains urgently unfinished.

There is also a reflexive argument. The deficiency narrative in health research, the framing of communities, patients and practitioners primarily in terms of what they lack, has been widely criticised for the ethical distortions it introduces and the research it discourages. This book takes that critique seriously and applies it to its own body of work: where the research has framed populations in terms of deficits rather than capacities, that framing is examined and its consequences acknowledged. Where the research has claimed influence that the evidence does not clearly support, that claim is revised. Where the gaps in the author's own methodology have been glossed over in the original publications, they are named here without deflection.

Structure and Methodology

Each chapter follows a three-part movement. The first part narrates the scientific story: the anchor publication, its institutional and intellectual context, the questions it was designed to answer and a fair account of what it found. The second part provides the critical reckoning: the gaps in methodology, the limitations the original paper acknowledged and those it did not, the distance between what the research demonstrated and what clinical practice required and an honest assessment of what the study failed to do. The third part is the Research Agenda Note: five open questions that the research programme points towards but has not answered, written not as a conventional literature review but as a genuine contribution to the scholarly conversation about what comes next.

Each chapter also includes an examination of the anchor publication's place in the subsequent literature. This is not a systematic review and does not claim to be one. It is a purposive reading of how the research entered the scholarly conversation after it appeared: where it was cited, in what contexts and what those citation patterns suggest about the field's engagement with the problem the original paper addressed. As the Preface notes, citations are imperfect evidence of impact. A paper can be cited opportunistically as background for a study that does not genuinely build on it, and a paper that changes clinical practice may receive fewer citations than a paper that generates methodological debate. What the citation record does allow, read carefully alongside the clinical and policy context, is a partial picture of whether the problems the research identified have been engaged with, confirmed, extended or quietly set aside. That partial picture is the best available evidence of scholarly influence, and this book uses it honestly, including where it is thin or ambiguous.

The research methodology for selecting anchor publications was straightforward. The author's full publication record was reviewed, and publications were grouped by research theme. Within each theme, the publication or cluster of publications that most fully represented the research programme's central contribution was selected as the anchor. In most cases this was a primary research paper; in one case, Chap. 11, it is an encyclopaedia entry, because the COVID-19 and medicines access work was conducted in a synthesising rather than empirical mode, and the genre difference itself is part of the story that chapter tells. In several cases, a cluster of related publications is treated together, because the intellectual contribution is distributed across papers that should be read as a sequence rather than as isolated studies.

A Note on Scope and Accountability

The relationship between published research and practice change is indirect and slow, and this book does not pretend otherwise. Practice change is mediated by institutional, regulatory, economic and professional factors that are largely outside the researcher's control. Where the research appears to have contributed to subsequent developments, including the development of validated instruments that subsequent researchers have used, the design of CPD programmes that built on documented deficiencies and the inclusion of regional findings in international systematic reviews and meta-analyses, those contributions are noted as evidence of scholarly engagement rather than proof of clinical impact. The honest position is that published research is a necessary but far from sufficient condition for practice change, and naming that limit honestly is part of the accountability this book owes its reader.

This book also does not claim to speak for collaborators. The research documented in these chapters was, in most cases, conducted by teams of investigators, graduate students and clinical colleagues whose contributions were real and indispensable. The retrospective judgements offered here are the author's own. Co-investigators who participated in the same studies may, entirely reasonably, reflect on them differently. Their perspectives are their own to express; this book expresses only the author's.

Readership

This book is written for pharmacy practice researchers, particularly those in the early stages of their careers, who are asking questions about how research programmes cohere and where their work might lead. It is written for pharmacy educators who are designing curricula and research training programmes and who want to understand how evidence from a sustained research programme can inform and reshape educational design. It is written for health services researchers in pharmacy and adjacent fields who are working on problems similar to those addressed here, and who may find value in an honest account of what approaches worked, what did not and what the evidence actually allows us to say. And it is written for the policymakers, professional bodies and pharmacy leaders who have the institutional authority to address the structural gaps that research can identify but research alone cannot close.

The gap between medicines and patients is not a research problem. It is a structural problem that research can illuminate. This book attempts to do that illuminating work with the rigour, honesty and professional accountability that the problem demands. Whether the illumination is acted on depends, as it always has, on those who hold the levers that research cannot reach.

Contents

Abbreviations

ACPE	Accreditation Council for Pharmacy Education
ACS	Acute coronary syndrome
AQLQ	Asthma Quality of Life Questionnaire
CCAPP	Canadian Council for Accreditation of Pharmacy Programs
CKD	Chronic kidney disease
COVID-19	Coronavirus disease 2019
CPD	Continuing professional development
FCTC	Framework Convention on Tobacco Control
HBM	Health belief model
HMC	Hamad Medical Corporation
JCEHP	Journal of Continuing Education in the Health Professions
LMQ	Living with Medicines Questionnaire
MENA	Middle East and North Africa
MRB	Medication-related burden
NAPRA	National Association of Pharmacy Regulatory Authorities
NCD	Non-communicable disease
PROMs	Patient-reported outcome measures
QNRF	Qatar National Research Fund
QRDI	Qatar Research, Development and Innovation
QU	Qatar University
RCT	Randomised Controlled Trial
TTM	Transtheoretical Model
UAE	United Arab Emirates
UREP	Undergraduate Research Experience Program
WHO	World Health Organization

Chapter 1
Pharmaceutical Care in the Middle East: A Reform That Arrived Before Its Infrastructure

1.1 The Anchor Publications

This chapter is built around four publications that together trace a sustained scholarly engagement with the same persistent question: why did a reform as intellectually compelling as pharmaceutical care make such limited headway in the Arabic-speaking Middle East, and what did the evidence actually show about the gap between what was being taught and what was being practised? The first, Kheir et al. (2008), published in the American Journal of Pharmaceutical Education, surveyed the status of pharmacy education and practice across 13 Middle Eastern countries and established the first comprehensive English-language baseline for the region. The second, Kheir et al. (2013), published in Avicenna, narrowed the lens to nine Arabic-speaking countries and examined pharmaceutical care implementation specifically, asking what was actually happening in practice when the philosophy was supposedly in operation. The third, Kheir (2013), a commentary in the International Journal of Clinical Pharmacy, identified a moment of grassroots professional energy that felt, briefly, like the beginning of genuine change. And the fourth, Awaisu et al. (2018), published in Pharmacy Education, compared the self-reported attitudes, perceived preparedness and identified barriers of final-year pharmacy students at Qatar University and Kuwait University toward pharmaceutical care, providing the first head-to-head cross-country comparison at the level of graduating students in the region. That final paper is the most intimate of the four: not the view from the policy landscape, but the view from the classroom, from students standing at the threshold between a curriculum that had prepared them to think like pharmaceutical care practitioners and a practice world they already suspected would not let them behave like one.

N. Kheir, *Medicines, Patients, and the Gaps Between*,
https://doi.org/10.1007/978-981-92-5395-1_1

1.2 The Idea and the Ground It Landed On

In 1990, Charles Hepler and Linda Strand published what would become one of the most cited papers in the history of pharmacy. Its argument was at once simple and radical. Pharmacy, they contended, had shed the apothecary role without yet finding a new professional identity commensurate with what pharmacists actually knew and could do. The solution was pharmaceutical care: the responsible provision of drug therapy for the purpose of achieving definite outcomes that improve a patient's quality of life (Hepler and Strand 1990). This was not a technical specification but a philosophical reorientation. It demanded that pharmacists stop organising their professional identity around the product they dispensed and start organising it around the patient they served, accepting accountability for outcomes, not just for process, and building cooperative relationships with patients and other health professionals that bore little resemblance to the transaction-based model that most community pharmacy, in most countries, was built around.

The paper landed differently in different parts of the world. In North America, it generated an immediate institutional response: the American Society of Health-System Pharmacists endorsed pharmaceutical care in 1992, the American Pharmacists Association followed, and major educational bodies began aligning curricula with the new philosophy. In Europe, the response was more measured but ultimately consequential, producing the Pharmaceutical Care Network Europe and regional implementation frameworks. But more than two decades after that seminal paper, the pharmaceutical care movement was still being described as a deferred dream, and even in countries with mature pharmacy systems, the translation from philosophy to daily practice had proven stubbornly incomplete. If the translation was difficult in well-resourced, institutionally stable health systems with established pharmacist-physician relationships and functioning remuneration frameworks, it was considerably more so in the Arabic-speaking Middle East, where none of those prerequisites could be taken for granted.

The Arabic-speaking world arrived at the pharmaceutical care conversation carrying the weight of a very different professional inheritance. Pharmacy in the Arab world has deep historical roots: the private apothecary in Baghdad around AD 750 is one of the earliest instances of pharmacy's independence from medicine, and the contributions of scholars such as Ibn Sina and al-Razi to pharmacology and therapeutics constitute an intellectual tradition that predates much of Western pharmaceutical science (Kheir et al. 2008). But historical eminence is not the same as contemporary professional infrastructure, and by the time pharmaceutical care arrived as a reform agenda, the region's pharmacy profession was, in most countries, still predominantly organised around dispensing in privately owned community pharmacies, with limited clinical training, fragmented regulatory oversight, and minimal institutional support for patient-centred practice.

1.3 What the 2008 Survey Found, and What It Could Not Find?

The survey of pharmacy education and practice across thirteen Middle Eastern countries, published in the American Journal of Pharmaceutical Education (Kheir et al. 2008), was not the first attempt to document pharmacy in the region, but it was the first to assemble a comparative, multicountry picture in a single peer-reviewed publication accessible to the international pharmacy research community. The methodology traded depth for breadth: information gathered through published literature, institutional websites and direct contact with programme or country representatives is vulnerable to the enthusiasms and blind spots of those who agree to participate. The paper acknowledged these limitations. In retrospect, they were more consequential than we allowed ourselves to say at the time.

What the survey found was a profession in the early stages of a transformation it had not yet equipped itself to complete. Seventy-eight active pharmacy schools in 12 countries were identified, admitting at least 14,000 students annually, with Egypt accounting for more than three-quarters of that intake (Kheir et al. 2008). Curricula were changing, with clinical pharmacy content appearing in syllabi previously dominated by pharmaceutical sciences, and a small number of countries beginning to introduce PharmD programmes. But the paper's own conclusion captured the central tension with a restraint that, looking back, understated the problem: while changes in pharmacy education had been relatively rapid over the prior decade, the advancement of pharmacy practice, particularly in the private sector, appeared to be slower (Kheir et al. 2008).

Slower is a relative term that does a good deal of work here. What the data actually showed was not a lag but a structural decoupling: two systems, education and practice, evolving at different rates and in response to different pressures, with no reliable mechanism for ensuring that what was taught would eventually be practised. Pharmacy schools were introducing pharmaceutical care into their curricula because international accreditation frameworks were beginning to require it, and because academic leaders understood that the profession's future demanded it. Community pharmacies were subject to no such pressure. Their economics were straightforward: revenue came from selling medicines, counselling attracted no additional payment, and time spent on a patient education conversation was time not spent on the next transaction. Hospital pharmacy was more advanced, as hospital pharmacists generally held postgraduate qualifications and operated within clinical structures that created some expectation of patient-centred work. But hospital pharmacy served a minority of the patient population. The community pharmacy, where the vast majority of patients collected their medicines, remained in most of the region a product-centred enterprise.

1.4 What the 2013 Paper Added: Naming the Structural Barriers?

Five years after the 2008 survey, we moved from description to analysis (Kheir et al. 2013). Using structured country informant reports, we examined not the educational landscape but the implementation reality: to what extent was pharmaceutical care actually being practised, in what settings, under what conditions, and with what constraints? The barriers identified were structural rather than personal. It was not that pharmacists lacked interest in pharmaceutical care or failed to understand its value. The informant reports suggested broad awareness of the philosophy and genuine aspiration toward its practice. What was missing were the conditions that make aspiration practicable: remuneration systems that rewarded dispensing and penalised the time patient consultation required; pharmacy laws that had not been updated to accommodate expanded pharmacist roles; postgraduate clinical training inaccessible to most practising pharmacists; and collaborative relationships with physicians, built on mutual recognition of each profession's clinical competence, that had not been established in most community or even hospital settings (Kheir et al. 2013).

There is a cruel irony embedded in this picture that the 2013 paper noted but perhaps did not press hard enough. The pharmaceutical care reforms were partly an educational project: change the curriculum, produce graduates who think like pharmaceutical care practitioners, and eventually practice will follow education, as though professional transformation were simply a matter of waiting long enough for the right graduates to accumulate. But the practice environments into which those graduates entered were not prepared to accommodate the fresh skills these graduates were bringing. A pharmacist trained to conduct a comprehensive medication review, to identify drug-related problems, to communicate therapeutic recommendations to a prescriber, steps into a community pharmacy expected to process a minimum of 40 prescriptions per shift, with no private consultation space, no prescriber relationship, and employer performance metrics that have nothing to do with patient outcomes. The training produced a professional identity the practice environment could not accommodate. The result was not the gradual transformation of practice but the gradual erosion of the newly trained pharmacist's professional aspirations, as the daily reality of the workplace shaped behaviour more powerfully than any curriculum could.

1.5 The Student's View: Evidence from the Classroom Floor

The most revealing evidence about the gap between pharmaceutical care education and practice did not come from surveys of the landscape or analyses of structural barriers. It came from the students themselves. A study we conducted with colleagues at Kuwait University, published in Pharmacy Education (Awaisu et al. 2018), was the first head-to-head comparison of self-reported attitudes, perceived preparedness and perceived barriers toward pharmaceutical care among final-year pharmacy students in two Gulf countries: Qatar University's College of Pharmacy (QU-CPH) and Kuwait University's Faculty of Pharmacy (KU-FoP). The study was, in a direct sense, an evaluation of the educational programmes my colleagues and I had helped to build at Qatar University, which gave its findings a particular personal and professional resonance.

The headline findings were encouraging. The vast majority of students from both universities expressed positive attitudes toward pharmaceutical care practice: 96.7% said they would like to perform pharmaceutical care as pharmacist practitioners, 95.1% agreed that pharmaceutical care is the right direction for the profession, and 100% agreed that providing pharmaceutical care would improve patients' health (Awaisu et al. 2018). These are not the numbers of a student cohort that has been inadequately educated in the philosophy of pharmaceutical care. They are the numbers of students who have genuinely internalised the mission. At QU-CPH, that internalisation had been achieved through a deliberately designed curriculum: pharmaceutical care principles introduced in the first professional year and threaded through subsequent years, problem-based and small-group learning formats, Objective Structured Clinical Examinations as performance assessments, and a Structured Practical Experience in Pharmacy comprising 960 h of experiential training across hospital, community and clinic rotations (Awaisu et al. 2018). The programme had received full accreditation from the Canadian Council for Accreditation of Pharmacy Programs for both its BSc and PharmD degrees, a standard that required demonstrable pharmaceutical care competency.

Alongside this, a Continuing Professional Development programme was developed at Qatar University that achieved the distinction of being the first such programme to receive accreditation from the Accreditation Council for Pharmacy Education outside the United States of America, a recognition that placed Qatar's pharmacy education infrastructure on an internationally benchmarked footing at a time when such standards were rarely applied in the region.

The findings beneath the headline, however, told a more complex story. Students perceived their preparedness as weakest in the administrative aspects of pharmaceutical care: the skills required to document care plans, manage service workflows, navigate institutional structures, and sustain a pharmaceutical care service over time. These are not peripheral competencies. They are the competencies that determine whether a pharmacist who understands pharmaceutical care philosophy can actually implement it in a real practice environment. Technical and communication skills were rated more highly, but administrative preparedness lagged consistently, a finding echoed in a 2002 US study and in earlier Kuwait-only data from 2014. The pattern was not unique to the Gulf; it reflected a widespread curricular tendency to teach the philosophy and clinical skills while underinvesting in the organisational and managerial competencies that practice change actually requires.

The barrier data were equally instructive, and pointed in directions that the structural analysis of Kheir et al. (2013) had already anticipated. Kuwait students identified lack of private counselling areas as their primary barrier, rated most significant by 76.9% of respondents. Qatar students identified organisational obstacles, specifically the absence of clear job descriptions for the pharmacist's expanded role, inadequate support from health authorities and weak collaboration among healthcare team members, rated significant by 66.6% (Awaisu et al. 2018). Kuwait students were also significantly more likely than Qatar students to identify poor professional image of the pharmacist in society as a major barrier (53.8% versus 4.8%, $p=0.001$). These are not the barriers of students who lack knowledge or motivation. They are the barriers of students who understand pharmaceutical care well enough to identify, precisely, the structural conditions that will prevent them from practising it, and who had not yet graduated.

The community pharmacy finding deserves particular emphasis, because it is, in its own quiet way, one of the most telling data points in this entire body of work. Not a single final-year student at Qatar University expressed a preference for community pharmacy as a future practice setting. Zero percent (Awaisu et al. 2018). Community pharmacy is exactly the setting where pharmaceutical care has the greatest potential population-level impact, where the largest number of patients collect their medicines, and where the unmet need for patient-centred medication management is most acute. And it was the setting that graduating pharmacists, trained explicitly to deliver pharmaceutical care, were least interested in entering. The reasons are not difficult to understand: students had observed community pharmacy practice during their rotations, and what they observed bore little resemblance to what their curriculum had described as the ideal. The dissonance between education and reality was strong enough to deflect career preferences toward hospital pharmacy, where pharmaceutical care was at least partially institutionalised. This is the structural decoupling described in Kheir et al. (2008), made visible not in aggregate data but in the individual career choices of sixty-three graduating students.

1.6 The Arab Pharmacy Spring: A Moment That Deserved More Analysis

In 2013, I published a commentary in which I pointed to something I was observing in the regional pharmacy community: a grassroots energy among younger pharmacists and pharmacy students that felt qualitatively different from the institutional rhetoric that had accompanied pharmaceutical care reform for two decades (Kheir 2013). Social media was amplifying voices that had previously had no platform. Students were organising discussions about what pharmacy could become rather than simply accepting what it was. I called it an Arab Pharmacy Spring, borrowing deliberately from the political language of the moment: the political uprisings of that era represented a grassroots rejection of structures that had long since exhausted their legitimacy, and something analogous seemed to be occurring, at a much smaller scale, within the pharmacy profession.

Whether that energy translated into sustained structural change is the honest question, and the literature does not provide a comfortable answer. A scoping review of pharmacy practice research across twelve Middle Eastern countries (Obaid et al. 2022) found that published research was still dominated by descriptive and cross-sectional designs, and still calling for implementation research that had not materialised.

A review of pharmaceutical care services in Middle Eastern countries covering 2013 to 2020, published in 2023, found that only a small fraction of published studies addressed barriers to implementation, and that the community pharmacy remained the least clinically transformed practice setting in the region. The spring, if it came, has not yet produced the institutional summer its advocates hoped for.

1.7 What the Field Did With These Publications?

The 2008 paper became, and has remained, the standard baseline reference for pharmacy practice and education research in the region. That it is still cited as foundational more than 15 years after its publication suggests that the subsequent evidence base has confirmed rather than superseded it. It was cited in UAE pharmacy education update letters, in competency-based education scoping reviews across the Eastern Mediterranean Region (Bajis et al. 2016), in comprehensive pharmacy practice scoping reviews covering twelve Middle Eastern countries (Obaid et al. 2022), and in clinical pharmacy development papers in Kuwait that explicitly described their findings as consistent with what Kheir et al. (2008) had documented. The 2013 Avicenna paper and commentary have been incorporated into subsequent analyses of implementation barriers and professional culture across the region. Awaisu et al. (2018) was cited in the systematic review by Boura et al. (2022) on pharmaceutical care education in the MENA region, which used the Qatar-Kuwait student comparison as one of the few available cross-country datasets at the student level, and in subsequent studies examining pharmacy student attitudes toward pharmaceutical care in Gulf countries.

What this citation trail reveals, read carefully, is not simply scholarly influence but the durability of the problem itself. Papers that cite Kheir et al. (2008) as a baseline are, in most cases, confirming that the baseline has not changed as much as the intervening years might have allowed. The education-practice gap documented in the mid-2000s was still being documented in the early 2020 s, in different countries and with different instruments, but with recognisably similar findings. This is not a failure of the researchers who cited the work. It is a finding about the nature of the structural problem: it is not amenable to correction by educational reform alone, and the profession has not yet mobilised the political, regulatory and economic levers that would be required to change it.

1.8 The Gap the Research Named but Could Not Close

All four publications were fundamentally diagnostic. They named the landscape with precision, identified the barriers with clarity and provided what the international literature had lacked: evidence from the Arabic-speaking Middle East itself, rather than inferences drawn from analogous settings elsewhere. What they could not do was change the structural conditions they described. A published survey does not reform a pharmacy law.

A student attitudes paper does not create private counselling spaces in community pharmacies, establish job descriptions for expanded pharmacist roles or persuade employers to accept the additional time that genuine patient consultation requires.

There is a version of this story in which the diagnostic publications were the necessary precondition for reform: you cannot fix what you have not named, and naming it in the peer-reviewed literature at least made it visible to those with the capacity to act. That version has some truth to it. But the critique levelled at descriptive health services research more generally, that it confirms what practitioners already know, produces findings filed and cited rather than acted upon, and benefits the academics who conduct it more than the patients whose circumstances it describes, deserves a direct response rather than deflection. The problem described in the 2008 and 2013 papers was already visible to every pharmacist practising in the region. And the graduating students of 2014, as Awaisu et al. (2018) documented, could already name the structural barriers before they had even entered practice. The research programme required courage of a different kind: not the courage to describe the problem, but the courage to follow it with implementation studies that tested specific interventions and measured their impact on what pharmacists actually did when a patient stood at the counter and asked for help.

1.9 Research Agenda Note

The research programme documented in this chapter points toward five open questions that represent the most important unfinished work on pharmaceutical care implementation in the Arabic-speaking Middle East.

First: which specific regulatory, remuneration and workforce reforms actually shift community pharmacy practice from a product-centred to a patient-centred model in Gulf health systems? The diagnostic literature, including the publications anchoring this chapter, has named the barriers repeatedly and consistently. What the field now needs is implementation research that treats jurisdictional variation across the Gulf as a natural experiment, comparing settings where reforms such as expanded scopes of practice or service-based remuneration have been introduced against settings where they have not, with counselling quality and patient outcomes as the endpoints.

Second: what happens to descriptive health services evidence after publication in this region, and why does it so rarely convert into structural change? The circularity documented in this chapter, in which new surveys confirm old surveys across two decades, is itself a researchable phenomenon. A study of the research-to-policy pathway in two or three Gulf states, tracing who reads the published evidence, which bodies cite it in policy documents, and where the translation chain breaks, would convert a source of professional frustration into an object of systematic inquiry.

Third: what became of the professional energy described as an Arab Pharmacy Spring, and under what institutional conditions does grassroots professional mobilisation in pharmacy produce durable organisational change? The 2013 commentary named a moment; no subsequent study has traced its trajectory. A historical and qualitative analysis of the professional associations, conferences and reform initiatives of that period, and of their institutional fate, would establish whether such moments require formal structures to outlast their founders.

Fourth: why has clinical pharmacy become institutionalised in the region's major hospital systems while community pharmacy has remained structurally static, and what does that divergence teach about the conditions of practice change? A comparative case study design, examining matched hospital and community settings within the same national systems, would isolate the governance, remuneration and accountability variables that differ between the two sectors and identify which of them are actionable.

Fifth: how do the aspirations of pharmacy graduates evolve once they enter the practice environments this chapter describes? The student preparedness evidence in Awaisu et al. (2018) established a baseline of positive attitudes at graduation. A longitudinal cohort study following graduates from Gulf pharmacy programmes across their first five years of practice, measuring the trajectory of their pharmaceutical care aspirations against the environments they enter, would document directly the education-environment gap that this book argues is structural.

1.10 What Remains?

The conditions identified across these four publications as prerequisites for genuine pharmaceutical care implementation remain, in most of the region, only partially in place. Some progress has been made: expanded pharmacist roles have been legislated in parts of the Gulf, clinical pharmacy services institutionalised in several major hospital systems, and the PharmD established as the standard entry-level qualification in a growing number of programmes. But the community pharmacy, where the majority of patient-pharmacist interactions occur and where the consequences of product-centred practice are most directly felt by patients, remains an environment that rewards dispensing speed over clinical engagement. A 2025 survey of community pharmacists across all seven emirates of the UAE found that pharmaceutical care was still less practised in community settings, that lack of time, insufficient staffing and workload pressure remained the primary perceived barriers, and that the structural conditions of practice had not substantially changed from what had been documented a decade and more earlier. The circularity of this finding, new data confirming old findings confirming older findings, is itself a commentary on the pace of change.

For students graduating now from pharmacy programmes in the Gulf, the situation described by Awaisu et al. (2018) has only partially improved. The curricula are better. The attitudes are positive. The barriers are largely the same. The community pharmacy still offers no private counselling space in most settings, no remuneration for pharmaceutical care services and no clear professional mandate for the kind of practice those students were trained to deliver. The pattern of career choices that the 2018 study documented, with graduates gravitating overwhelmingly toward hospital pharmacy, postgraduate study, academia and government institutions, and virtually none choosing community pharmacy, has persisted. It is not a reflection of poor graduate quality or inadequate professional ambition. As argued in a recent analysis of community pharmacy in low- and middle-income countries, community pharmacies in these settings are widely accessible yet underutilised, because regulatory constraints, poor remuneration, limited professional development opportunities and a practice environment that contradicts what graduates were trained to do make community pharmacy professionally untenable for well-educated pharmacists who have options (Kheir 2025). Qatar's community pharmacy sector, characterised by ownership structures that prioritise commercial throughput, workforce conditions that offer pharmacists minimal clinical autonomy and regulatory frameworks that have not kept pace with professional education, represents a specific and well-documented instance of this general problem (Kheir 2016).

Until the structural conditions change, education will continue to produce graduates whose aspirations the practice environment systematically disappoints, and the pharmacy profession in the Arab Middle East will continue to promise its patients a standard of care it does not yet have the infrastructure to deliver. The community pharmacy, the most accessible point of pharmaceutical care for the largest number of patients, will continue to be the setting that the profession's best-trained graduates are least willing to enter. That is the most important unresolved finding of this entire body of work.[1]

References

Awaisu A, Katoue MG, Al-Taweel D, Bacha R, El-Gargawi A, Kheir N (2018) Self-reported attitudes and perceived preparedness to provide pharmaceutical care among final year pharmacy students in Qatar and Kuwait. Pharm Educ 18(1):284–291*

Bajis D, Chaar B, Penm J, Moles R (2016) Competency-based pharmacy education in the Eastern Mediterranean Region: a scoping review. Curr Pharm Teach Learn 8(3):401–428

Boura F, Awaisu A, ElGeed H, Katoue M, Kheir N (2022) Pharmaceutical care education at pharmacy colleges in the Middle East and North Africa region: a systematic review. J Clin Pharm Ther 47(8):1134–1148*

Hepler CD, Strand LM (1990) Opportunities and responsibilities in pharmaceutical care. Am J Hosp Pharm 47(3):533–543

Kheir N (2013) An Arab pharmacy spring: taking matters in their own hands. Int J Clin Pharm 35(5):665–667*

Kheir N (2016) Pharmacy practice in Qatar. In: Babar ZUD (ed) Pharmacy practice in developing countries: achievements and challenges. Academic Press/Elsevier, pp 233–252*

Kheir N (2025) The paradox of community pharmacy practice in low- and middle-income countries (LMICs). J Pharm Policy Pract 18(1):2475082*

Kheir N, Al Saad D, Al Naimi S (2013) Pharmaceutical care in the Arabic-speaking Middle East: literature review and country informant feedback. Avicenna 2013(2) *

Kheir N, Zaidan M, Younes H, El Hajj M, Wilbur K, Jewesson PJ (2008) Pharmacy education and practice in 13 Middle Eastern countries. Am J Pharm Educ 72(6):133*

Obaid D, El-Dahiyat F, Babar ZUD (2022) Pharmacy practice and clinical pharmacy research in the Middle East: a scoping review of studies from Bahrain, Iraq, Jordan, Kuwait, Lebanon, Oman, Palestine, Qatar, Saudi Arabia, Syria, United Arab Emirates, and Yemen. J Pharm Policy Pract 15(1):40

[1] Publications by the author of this book are marked with an asterisk (*) in references.

Chapter 2
The Patient Behind the Prescription: Medication-Related Burden, What We Learned, and What We Have Not Yet Changed

2.1 The Anchor Publications

This chapter is built around four publications that, taken together, represent a sustained research programme on medication-related burden in Qatar. The first, Zidan et al. (2016a), translated and culturally adapted the Living with Medicines Questionnaire (LMQ) into Arabic, providing the measurement infrastructure on which the subsequent clinical studies depended. The second, Zidan et al. (2018), used the Arabic LMQ to assess medication-related burden among patients with non-communicable diseases attending primary healthcare clinics in Qatar, and investigated the relationship between that burden and medication adherence. The third, Al-Mansouri et al. (2021), assessed treatment burden and quality of life in chronic kidney disease patients at Fahad Bin Jassim Kidney Center, using the Treatment Burden Questionnaire alongside the Kidney Disease Quality of Life instrument. And the fourth, Zidan et al. (2016b), established the protocol for the ACS randomised controlled trial at Heart Hospital, Hamad Medical Corporation, the first RCT of its kind in the Gulf cardiovascular setting, which sought to determine whether a structured pharmacist-delivered intervention at discharge and post-discharge could improve medication adherence and reduce readmission in post-ACS patients. Reading these publications in sequence reveals not simply a series of independent studies, but a coherent intellectual trajectory: from instrument development, through prevalence and correlation studies, toward a controlled clinical test of whether measurement of burden and pharmacist intervention could actually change patient outcomes.

N. Kheir, *Medicines, Patients, and the Gaps Between*,
https://doi.org/10.1007/978-981-92-5395-1_2

2.2 Reframing Non-Adherence: From Failure to Rational Response

Non-adherence to prescribed medication regimens is one of the most extensively studied and most persistently intractable problems in health services research. The epidemiological picture has been stable for decades: approximately half of patients with chronic conditions do not take their medications as prescribed, and the clinical and economic consequences, measured in disease progression, preventable hospitalisations, and avoidable mortality, are substantial (Sabaté 2003). The research response has been equally extensive, producing a literature of considerable breadth on the patient-level, provider-level and system-level correlates of non-adherence, and generating a wide range of interventions, from reminder systems and simplified packaging to motivational interviewing and pharmacist-led counselling, each of which shows modest effects in specific populations under controlled conditions.

What this literature has been slower to produce is a patient-centred reframing of the question itself. The adherence framework, as traditionally applied, positions non-adherence as a failure, whether of the patient's motivation, knowledge or self-efficacy, or of the clinician's communication, or of the healthcare system's structural support. What it does not adequately capture is the possibility that non-adherence is, in many cases, a rational response by a person managing an unreasonable workload. A patient prescribed 12 medications, attending dialysis three times a week, adjusting diet and fluid intake, managing side effects and navigating the logistical demands of multiple clinic appointments is not failing to adhere because she does not understand the importance of her medications. She is prioritising, negotiating and making decisions in a context of finite time, energy and resources. The aggregate demand of the treatment regimen, what researchers have come to call treatment burden or medication-related burden, is itself a clinically significant determinant of how patients engage with their care (Tran et al. 2012; Sav et al. 2013).

Treatment burden, defined as the workload of self-managing one's health and the impact of that workload on patient functioning and wellbeing, gained formal conceptual traction in the early 2010s, when Tran, Montori, Ravaud and colleagues published a foundational framework and measurement instrument, and May and colleagues articulated the theoretical structure of what they called Burden of Treatment Theory (Tran et al. 2012). The theory describes a balance between the demands imposed by treatment, including medication management, appointment attendance, lifestyle modification and health monitoring, and the patient's capacity to meet those demands, which varies with cognitive resources, social support, financial circumstances and co-existing life obligations. When demands exceed capacity, patients adapt: they skip doses, miss appointments, simplify regimens informally and decline new treatments. These adaptations are not failures. They are rational. But they carry clinical risks that the healthcare system, focused on the treatment it prescribed rather than the life it disrupted, often fails to recognise or address.

The Qatar research programme documented in this chapter was grounded in this reframing from the outset. It asked not simply how burdensome patients found their treatment, but what the relationship between that burden and their clinical behaviour was, and whether healthcare providers had the instruments and the mandate to do anything about it. The foundational step was measurement.

2.3 Building the Measurement Infrastructure: The Arabic LMQ

No measurement programme can proceed without a valid instrument. The Living with Medicines Questionnaire (LMQ), developed originally in English by Krska and colleagues, is a patient-reported measure of medication-related burden whose current version comprises 41 items across eight domains, including relationships with health professionals, practical difficulties, interference with daily life, effectiveness, side effects and autonomy (Krska et al. 2017; Katusiime et al. 2018). It captures, with more granularity than most burden instruments, the patient's subjective experience of living with a complex medication regimen over time. Its limitation, for the Qatar context, was obvious: it existed only in English, and the patient population in Qatar's primary care settings is predominantly Arabic-speaking, with substantial linguistic and cultural heterogeneity across the various dialects and educational backgrounds that characterise the population.

Our research group at Qatar University's College of Pharmacy addressed this directly, undertaking the translation and cultural adaptation of the LMQ into Arabic following the International Society for Pharmacoeconomics and Outcomes Research guidelines for patient-reported outcome translation (Zidan et al. 2016a). The process involved forward translation, synthesis, back-translation, expert committee review and cognitive debriefing with Arabic-speaking patients, each step designed to ensure that the translated instrument captured the same constructs as the original rather than merely converting its words. This kind of foundational methodological work is unglamorous in the economy of academic publishing. It does not generate striking clinical findings, and it does not attract the same citation volumes as intervention trials. But it is indispensable: without a validated Arabic instrument, all subsequent measurement of medication-related burden in Arabic-speaking populations would have relied on tools of unverified validity, producing data of uncertain interpretive value. The Arabic LMQ created the methodological platform on which the clinical studies that followed were built.

The impact of this contribution has been acknowledged in the literature. A 2024 paper describing the development of a new Arabic medication-related burden quality of life tool noted that three existing measures of treatment burden had been translated into Arabic, of which the LMQ was one, while also identifying limitations in the existing instruments, including the length of the LMQ at 41 items, that subsequent instrument developers would need to address (Al-Ebrahim et al. 2024). This is the normal productive cycle of measurement science: a translation opens a field of inquiry, subsequent researchers apply the tool, identify its limitations in specific populations and develop refinements. The Arabic LMQ initiated that cycle in the Middle East context.

2.4 Medication-Related Burden in Primary Care: What the NCD Study Found?

The Arabic LMQ was subsequently deployed in a cross-sectional study of 293 patients with diabetes, with or without comorbidities, attending three primary healthcare clinics in Qatar (Zidan et al. 2018). The majority, 66.8%, reported minimal medication-related burden, while 24.1% reported moderate burden and a small proportion reported severe burden. These figures require careful interpretation: they might initially appear reassuring, but the threshold effects embedded in any scale of this kind mean that a patient reporting minimal burden may still be experiencing a degree of disruption to daily life that, while below the threshold for clinical concern on a population level, is clinically significant for that individual. More importantly, the study found a statistically significant positive correlation between LMQ scores and scores on the Adherence to Refills and Medications Scale, with a Spearman correlation coefficient of 0.317 ($p < 0.0005$). Higher burden was associated with lower adherence. This was not surprising, but it was, in the Qatar context, the first time it had been demonstrated quantitatively, and the precision of the demonstration matters.

The study's design had a methodological limitation that its authors acknowledged and that deserves direct reflection here. A cross-sectional correlation cannot establish causation. The association between higher LMQ scores and lower adherence is consistent with the hypothesis that burden causes non-adherence, but it is equally consistent with the hypothesis that non-adherent patients, who by definition have a more conflicted relationship with their medications, perceive those medications as more burdensome, or that a third variable, such as disease severity or socioeconomic constraint, drives both. Longitudinal studies, preferably with intervention arms, are needed to establish whether reducing burden improves adherence, and those studies have not yet been conducted in the Qatar primary care context. The correlation finding was a necessary first step. It was not the last step, and it has not yet been followed by the implementation research it implies.

2.5 Treatment Burden in Chronic Kidney Disease: The Dialysis Study

Al-Mansouri et al. (2021) addressed a clinically distinct but conceptually related question in a patient population for whom the burden of treatment is, almost by definition, extreme. Chronic kidney disease in its advanced stages, particularly when managed by haemodialysis, imposes demands on patients that are qualitatively different from those faced by patients managing oral medications in primary care. Haemodialysis requires attendance at a dialysis centre three times per week for sessions lasting 3–5 h, during which the patient is physically connected to a machine, often fatigued, and unable to engage in normal daily activities. Between sessions, patients manage strict fluid and dietary restrictions, a complex oral medication regimen typically comprising multiple phosphate binders, antihypertensives, erythropoiesis-stimulating agents and other agents, and the psychological weight of a condition that is life-limiting and progressive. The treatment burden in this population is not a concern at the margins. It is a central feature of the patient's life.

The study enrolled 280 CKD patients at Fahad Bin Jassim Kidney Center in Qatar, 223 on haemodialysis and 57 in the pre-dialysis stage, and assessed treatment burden using the Treatment Burden Questionnaire alongside health-related quality of life measured by the Kidney Disease Quality of Life instrument. The findings confirmed, with quantitative precision in the Qatari context, what the international literature had suggested: haemodialysis patients experienced significantly higher treatment burden than pre-dialysis patients, medication burden and treatment-imposed lifestyle changes were the highest perceived sources of burden, and there was a strong negative correlation between treatment burden and health-related quality of life scores. Patients who were divorced or widowed, unemployed, or less educated reported significantly higher burden, a pattern pointing directly to the social determinants of the treatment experience that clinical management in Qatar had not systematically addressed (Al-Mansouri et al. 2021).

A companion conference presentation, delivered in 2019 before the full paper was published, had already flagged the scale of the polypharmacy problem in this cohort: patients were prescribed a median of 12 oral medications and three parenteral medications, placing their pill burden among the highest documented in the regional renal care literature at that time. Twelve oral medications, taken daily, with timing constraints around dialysis sessions, dietary restrictions on certain formulations, and potential interactions with the dialysate and with each other, represent a management challenge that most clinical guidelines, written around single-condition pharmacotherapy, are not designed to address. The finding was not a statistical artefact. It was a description of reality.

The international literature on CKD treatment burden provides important context for the Qatar findings. A 2023 systematic review and meta-analysis of health-related quality of life in CKD patients in low- and lower-middle-income countries found that the transition from pre-dialysis to dialysis was associated with a substantial worsening in perceived disease burden across multiple instruments, and that the HRQoL deficits observed in these settings were substantially greater than those reported in high-income country cohorts, likely reflecting the compounding effects of inadequate symptom control, financial hardship and limited social support infrastructure. Qatar is not a low-income country, but the patient population at Fahad Bin Jassim Kidney Center is predominantly composed of low-income migrant workers for whom the financial and social dimensions of treatment burden carry particular weight. The finding that unemployment and lower educational attainment were associated with higher burden reflects the intersection of clinical complexity with economic vulnerability in a way that straightforward clinical management cannot address without attending to the social circumstances of the patient.

2.6 The ACS Protocol: Establishing the Research Question

A programme of research designed and conducted with colleagues at Heart Hospital, Hamad Medical Corporation, sought to test directly whether pharmacist intervention could improve outcomes in post-ACS patients. The protocol, published in BMJ Open (Zidan et al. 2016b), was the first registered RCT of its kind in the Gulf cardiovascular setting. The clinical urgency was clear: cardiovascular disease was the leading cause of morbidity and mortality in Qatar, with 16,736 ACS admissions recorded between 1991 and 2010 at Hamad Medical Corporation (Zidan et al. 2016b), and fewer than 80% of ACS patients were using the recommended quadruple secondary prevention therapy after discharge. The evidence base for this combination therapy is unambiguous: adherence to secondary prevention medications after ACS significantly reduces the risk of subsequent cardiovascular events, and the gap between recommended and actual use translates directly into preventable morbidity and mortality.

The three-arm trial design compared standard care against pharmacist-delivered medication reconciliation and counselling at discharge, and against a combined pharmacist and patient education intervention with tailored follow-up post-discharge. The protocol publication established the trial's existence, design and hypotheses in the peer-reviewed literature, enabling methodological scrutiny and contributing to the visibility of Gulf-based pharmaceutical care research internationally. In a research environment where the Gulf is substantially underrepresented in the international pharmacy literature, a registered and published protocol establishes credibility for the research programme and makes it citable by others working in similar settings.

The trial was completed, and its outcomes were subsequently addressed in a quasi-experimental study by El Hajj et al. (2023), conducted at the same Heart Hospital in Qatar and explicitly citing Zidan et al. (2016b) as its direct precursor. That study found that a structured pharmacist-delivered intervention for post-ACS patients was associated with significant reductions in all-cause hospitalisation and cardiac-related readmissions at 6 months post-discharge (El Hajj et al. 2023). The result is consistent with the international evidence base: a systematic review by Weeda and colleagues (2023) found that pharmacist-driven transitions of care interventions were associated with numerically lower readmission rates and more favourable secondary prevention measures and adherence, though the authors appropriately noted that sufficiently powered studies were still required to confirm these benefits definitively. The Qatar evidence adds a regionally specific data point to that international picture.

2.7 What the Field Did With These Publications?

The citation trail for this cluster of publications reveals a pattern common in clinical pharmacy research: foundational methodological work attracts modest but steady citation as subsequent researchers use or adapt the instrument; observational studies attract citations from researchers confirming or extending the findings in related populations and protocol publications attract citations both from subsequent outcome publications and from researchers in related fields who use the design as a methodological reference point.

The Arabic LMQ (Zidan et al. 2016a) has been cited in burden studies across Qatar and the wider region, and in Arabic-language PRO measurement scoping reviews that acknowledge it as one of the three available Arabic treatment burden instruments. The primary care NCD study (Zidan et al. 2018) has been cited in subsequent regional NCD adherence research and in papers calling for greater pharmacist involvement in primary care chronic disease management, where the correlation between burden and adherence provides a compelling clinical rationale for intervention. Both papers were cited together in a Frontiers in Pharmacology study on medication-related burden and adherence, which explicitly acknowledged their role in establishing the Arabic-language measurement framework for this field of inquiry.

Zidan et al. (2016b) has been cited in a systematic review of pharmacist-involved care for patients with heart failure and ACS (Lau et al. 2021), in Pharmacy Times clinical guidance on ACS management, and in regional health literacy research examining what post-ACS patients understood about their secondary prevention regimen. Al-Mansouri et al. (2021) has been cited in subsequent regional CKD research and in advocacy documents for greater pharmacist involvement in renal care management, where the treatment burden data provide a compelling clinical rationale for pharmacist-led medication review and burden assessment in the dialysis setting.

2.8 From Research to the Classroom: Theoretical Frameworks for Burden-Sensitive Care

The impact of this research programme was not confined to the peer-reviewed literature or to subsequent clinical studies. It also shaped, in a direct and deliberate way, how the next generation of pharmacists in Qatar was taught to think about the relationship between patients and their medications. This connection between research findings and educational design is one of the less visible but most durable forms of scholarly impact, and it deserves to be named explicitly.

As part of the foundational curriculum of the newly established College of Pharmacy at Qatar University, a course titled Pharmacy and Healthcare was developed and delivered to first-year pharmacy students across two semesters. Within this course, and within the accompanying Professional Skills course delivered in the second semester, two behaviour change frameworks were introduced and taught in deliberate combination: the Transtheoretical Model of Change (TTM) and the Health Belief Model (HBM). Each framework was well-established in the health behaviour literature; what was pedagogically distinctive was the way they were presented not as alternative theories but as complementary tools for a single clinical problem, and the sequence in which their application was taught.

The TTM, developed by Prochaska and DiClemente in the early 1980s, conceptualises health behaviour change as a staged process rather than a discrete event (Prochaska and DiClemente 1983). The model identifies five stages through which individuals typically move when modifying a health-related behaviour: precontemplation, in which the person has no intention to change in the foreseeable future; contemplation, in which they are aware that a problem exists and are seriously thinking about changing but have not yet committed to action; preparation, in which they intend to take action and may have begun taking small steps; action, in which they are actively modifying their behaviour; and maintenance, in which they work to sustain the change and prevent relapse. The model has been widely applied in clinical contexts ranging from smoking cessation to medication adherence, and it had particular relevance to the patient populations that the Qatar burden research had been studying: patients whose high treatment burden had left them stuck in precontemplation or at best contemplation, making no visible progress toward better adherence not because they lacked information but because the aggregate demands of their treatment regimen had exhausted their capacity to change.

The HBM, first formulated by Rosenstock and colleagues in the 1950s to explain why people failed to participate in disease prevention programmes, proposes that individuals take health-related action based on a specific set of perceptual factors: their perceived susceptibility to a health threat, their perceived severity of the consequences of that threat, their perceived benefits of taking action, the perceived barriers that would prevent them from acting, cues to action that trigger the behaviour, and their self-efficacy, their confidence that they can successfully perform the required behaviour (Rosenstock 1974). Where the TTM describes the stages of change, the HBM explains the beliefs that determine whether and why a person moves between those stages.

The pedagogical argument made in the classroom was precisely this: that the TTM and HBM are most powerful when used together, in sequence, and that the sequence matters enormously. Most clinical behaviour change training focuses on the action and maintenance stages of the TTM, the territory in which pharmacists feel most confident because the patient has already committed to change and is asking for support in sustaining it. But the patients who are hardest to reach, and who contribute most to the burden of non-adherence in chronic disease populations, are not in the action stage. They are in precontemplation. They are not asking for help because they do not yet believe that change is possible, necessary, or relevant to them.

The teaching advanced a specific clinical logic: before a pharmacist can help a patient in precontemplation move toward contemplation, they must first understand why that patient is not yet contemplating change. The HBM provides the diagnostic framework for that understanding. A patient who smokes, for example, and shows no intention of stopping, is not simply unmotivated. They may perceive their susceptibility to smoking-related harm as low, because they have smoked for 30 years without a heart attack and know people who have done the same. They may perceive the barriers to cessation as prohibitively high, because every previous attempt has ended in relapse. They may have low self-efficacy for quitting, not because they lack willpower but because their previous attempts have not been supported by adequate clinical intervention. Each of these perceptual configurations requires a different pharmacist response. Only by identifying which specific beliefs are keeping the patient in precontemplation can the pharmacist design an intervention that genuinely moves them toward contemplation, rather than simply repeating information that has already failed to produce change.

This teaching emerged directly from the research documented in this chapter. The burden studies had shown, with quantitative precision, that high medication-related burden was associated with lower adherence. But a burden score, however, precisely measured, does not tell the pharmacist what to do next. The TTM tells the pharmacist where the patient is in the change process. The HBM tells the pharmacist why the patient is there. Together, they equip the pharmacist not just to measure the problem but to intervene in it intelligently. That clinical logic, developed through research and refined through practice, was what was placed in front of first-year pharmacy students at Qatar University, in the conviction that the foundational professional formation of a pharmacist should include not only knowledge of drug mechanisms and disease management, but a theoretically grounded understanding of why patients do what they do, and what the pharmacist can realistically do about it.

The inclusion of these frameworks in the first-year curriculum at a school that had received CCAPP accreditation and whose CPD programme had achieved ACPE accreditation outside the United States represented a deliberate educational philosophy: that patient behaviour is not a residual problem to be managed after pharmacotherapy is optimised, but a central clinical variable that pharmacists must be trained to understand and engage with from the earliest stages of their professional formation. That philosophy was not arrived at abstractly. It was the direct educational consequence of research that had spent years measuring the distance between what patients were prescribed and what they actually took, and asking why.

2.9 The Gap the Research Left Open

The most significant limitation of this research programme is the gap between measurement and intervention. Considerable effort was invested in demonstrating that treatment burden was real, measurable and associated with clinically significant outcomes in multiple patient populations. What none of these studies did, within their scope as designed, was test what happens when healthcare providers systematically address burden as part of clinical care. That translational step, from measuring burden to acting on it in a way that changes patient outcomes, is where the research programme remains incomplete.

The cross-sectional designs of the LMQ and CKD studies capture prevalence and correlation, not trajectory or causation. Treatment burden is not a static property of a patient or a regimen. It evolves as disease progresses, as medications accumulate, as social circumstances change, and as the patient's own capacity to manage the workload fluctuates with age, employment and family circumstances. A patient who reports minimal burden at one assessment may report severe burden 12 months later following the addition of a new medication or the loss of a supporting family member. Longitudinal studies would have told a richer and more actionable story, and their absence is a genuine limitation of what this body of work can recommend to clinicians.

A second gap concerns the social determinants identified in the CKD study. The finding that divorced or widowed, unemployed and less educated patients reported significantly higher burden is clinically important. But identifying the social correlates of burden and addressing them are different things, and the clinical infrastructure for addressing social determinants of treatment burden in Qatar's renal care system, including social work support, flexible appointment scheduling, financial assistance for medication costs and caregiver engagement programmes, did not exist in a form adequate to the problem at the time of the study. Whether it has developed since is a question the literature has not yet systematically addressed.

There is also a gap between the theoretical frameworks taught in the classroom and their systematic application in clinical practice. The TTM and HBM were introduced to first-year pharmacy students at Qatar University as tools for understanding and addressing the kind of non-adherence that burden research had characterised. Whether graduates of that programme applied those frameworks in their subsequent clinical practice, whether the theoretical training translated into different patient conversations and different clinical decisions, is an outcomes question that has not been formally evaluated. Curriculum design and clinical behaviour change are both long-horizon investments, and the evidence of their impact is correspondingly slow to accumulate.

2.10 Research Agenda Note

The burden research programme documented in this chapter points toward five open questions that represent the most important unfinished work on medication-related burden in the region and beyond.

First: does burden-sensitive pharmaceutical care improve patient outcomes compared with usual care? The instruments now exist in Arabic, and the association between burden and non-adherence has been established in Qatari primary care. The decisive next study is a pragmatic trial in which pharmacists routinely assess, discuss and respond to patients' reported treatment burden within existing clinic workflow, with adherence, clinical control and quality of life as endpoints, operationalising the Minimally Disruptive Medicine philosophy in a Middle Eastern care setting.

Second: what is the longitudinal trajectory of medication-related burden as disease progresses and life circumstances change? The cross-sectional designs of the studies anchoring this chapter capture prevalence and correlation, not evolution. Cohort studies that follow patients across medication additions, transitions to dialysis, and changes in employment and family support would identify the inflection points at which burden escalates and at which intervention is most likely to help.

Third: how should burden-reducing care be designed for economically and socially vulnerable patients, such as the low-income migrant workers who predominate in Qatar's dialysis population? The CKD study found that unemployment and lower educational attainment were associated with higher burden. Intervention research that pairs clinical burden assessment with practical supports addressing the social dimensions of treatment workload has not been attempted in this population and is overdue.

Fourth: what is the minimal burden measure that is clinically useful in routine practice? The research instruments are long by design; a busy clinic requires something shorter that preserves validity. Building on the Arabic LMQ and the subsequent Arabic MRB-QoL work, a programme of psychometric reduction and clinical utility testing would produce the screening tool that routine burden-sensitive care requires.

Fifth: can aggregated burden data function as a health system indicator? If burden scores were collected routinely across clinics, they could inform formulary decisions, deprescribing programmes and service design in the same way that adherence and readmission data now do. Whether aggregate patient-reported burden is stable, interpretable, and actionable at the system level is an empirical question no health system has yet tested.

2.11 What Remains?

The medication-related burden framework has genuine transformative potential for pharmaceutical care in the Middle East, but only if it is connected to clinical practice change rather than used solely as a research outcome. The instruments now exist in Arabic. The association between burden and non-adherence has been established in the primary care context in Qatar. The scale of burden in the CKD dialysis population has been quantified. The pharmacist-delivered ACS intervention has demonstrated reduced readmissions at the same institution. What is missing is the systematic integration of burden assessment into routine clinical workflow across these patient populations, and the implementation research to test whether burden-sensitive pharmaceutical care, in which pharmacists routinely assess, discuss and respond to patients' reported treatment burden, produces better outcomes than care as usual.

The Minimally Disruptive Medicine framework, developed by Montori and colleagues at the Mayo Clinic, offers one model for how this might be operationalised: a clinical philosophy in which treatment plans are explicitly designed to fit the patient's life rather than requiring the patient's life to accommodate the treatment (Montori et al. 2013). Pharmaceutical care, properly understood, is philosophically aligned with this approach, and the pharmacist is, in the healthcare team, the professional best positioned to identify where treatment regimens have become disruptive and to initiate the clinical conversations that would allow them to be rationalised. The TTM and HBM, taught to first-year pharmacy students in Qatar as a framework for understanding why patients do not change, provide the clinical language for those conversations. Building the evidence that pharmacist-led burden-sensitive care works, in the specific healthcare settings of the Gulf and wider Middle East, is the most important task remaining from this body of work. It is also, nearly a decade after the LMQ translation was published, still largely undone.[1]

[1]Publications by the author of this book are marked with an asterisk (*) in references.

References

Al-Ebrahim SQ, Harrison J, Chen TF, Alzubaidi H, Mohammed MA (2024) The Arabic medication-related burden quality of life (MRB-QoL) tool: cross-cultural adaptation and content validation. Explor Res Clin Soc Pharm 16:100523

Al-Mansouri A, Al-Ali FS, Hamad AI, Mohamed Ibrahim MI, Kheir N, Ibrahim RA, AlBakri M, Awaisu A (2021) Assessment of treatment burden and its impact on quality of life in dialysis-dependent and pre-dialysis chronic kidney disease patients. Res Soc Adm Pharm 17(11):1937–1944*

El Hajj MS, Kaddoura R, Abu Yousef SEA, Orabi B, Awaisu A, AlYafei S, Shami R, Mahfoud ZR (2023) Effectiveness of a structured pharmacist-delivered intervention for patients post-acute coronary syndromes on all-cause hospitalizations and cardiac-related hospital readmissions: a prospective quasi-experimental study. Int J Clin Pharm 45(3):630–640

Katusiime B, Corlett SA, Krska J (2018) Development and validation of a revised instrument to measure burden of long-term medicines use: the Living with Medicines Questionnaire version 3. Patient Relat Outcome Meas 9:155–168

Krska J, Katusiime B, Corlett SA (2017) Validation of an instrument to measure patients' experiences of medicine use: the Living with Medicines Questionnaire. Patient Prefer Adherence 11:671–679

Lau WCY et al (2021) Pharmacist-involved care for patients with heart failure and acute coronary syndrome: a systematic review with qualitative and quantitative meta-analysis. Br J Clin Pharmacol 87(10):3761–3782

Montori VM, Brito JP, Murad MH (2013) The optimal practice of evidence-based medicine: incorporating patient preferences in practice guidelines. JAMA 310(23):2503–2504

Prochaska JO, DiClemente CC (1983) Stages and processes of self-change of smoking: toward an integrative model of change. J Consult Clin Psychol 51(3):390–395

Rosenstock IM (1974) Historical origins of the health belief model. Health Educ Monogr 2(4):328–335

Sabaté E (2003) Adherence to long-term therapies: evidence for action. World Health Organization, Geneva

Sav A, Kendall E, McMillan SS et al (2013) You say treatment, I say hard work': treatment burden among people with chronic illness and their carers in Australia. Health Soc Care Community 21(6):665–674

Tran VT, Montori VM, Eton DT, Baruch D, Falissard B, Ravaud P (2012) Development and description of measurement properties of an instrument to assess treatment burden among patients with multiple chronic conditions. BMC Med 10:68

Zidan A, Awaisu A, El-Hajj MS, Al-Abdulla SA, Figueroa DCR, Kheir N (2018) Medication-related burden among patients with chronic disease conditions: perspectives of patients attending non-communicable disease clinics in a primary healthcare setting in Qatar. Pharmacy 6(3):85 (Kheir senior author) *

Zidan A, Awaisu A, Hasan S, Kheir N (2016a) The Living with Medicines Questionnaire: translation and cultural adaptation into the Arabic context. Value Health Reg Issues 10:36–40. (Kheir senior author)*

Zidan A, Awaisu A, Kheir N, Mahfoud Z, Kaddoura R, AlYafei S, El Hajj MS (2016b) Impact of a pharmacist-delivered discharge and follow-up intervention for patients with acute coronary syndromes in Qatar: a study protocol for a randomised controlled trial. BMJ Open 6(11):e012141*

Chapter 3
Measuring What Matters: Quality of Life and the New Zealand Pharmaceutical Care Experience

3.1 The Anchor Publications

This chapter is built around four publications arising from a doctoral research programme conducted at the School of Pharmacy, University of Otago, Dunedin and the broader Otago/Southland Comprehensive Pharmaceutical Care Asthma Project with which it was associated. In order of publication, these are: Kheir et al. (2001), which reported the health-related quality of life outcomes of the pharmaceutical care service for patients with asthma in the Otago and Southland regions of New Zealand's South Island; Emmerton et al. (2003), which documented the full implementation and clinical outcomes of the demonstration project; Kheir et al. (2004), which situated quality of life measurement within the broader philosophical framework of pharmaceutical care; and Kheir et al. (2008a), which assessed the psychometric responsiveness of the Asthma Quality of Life Questionnaire in the pharmaceutical care context. Together, these four papers represent a cluster of evidence that addressed a question the New Zealand pharmacy profession was asking at a specific and historically significant moment: if pharmaceutical care was to be taken seriously as a patient-centred reform, could it be shown, with rigour, to improve the quality of patients' lives?

3.2 Arriving in Otago: A Profession at a Crossroads

When I arrived in New Zealand in the late 1990s to pursue my PhD at the School of Pharmacy, University of Otago, I entered an institution and a professional environment that was, in certain respects, ahead of the international curve. New Zealand had, by the mid-1990s, embraced pharmaceutical care with an enthusiasm that few other countries could match. As Kheir et al. (2001) noted at the time, New Zealand had by that point probably the largest number of pharmaceutical care-trained pharmacists

N. Kheir, *Medicines, Patients, and the Gaps Between*,
https://doi.org/10.1007/978-981-92-5395-1_3

per capita in the world, a remarkable statistic that reflected a genuine professional commitment to the Hepler-Strand vision (Hepler and Strand 1990). Pharmaceutical care services had begun to be recognised in New Zealand in the mid-1990s, but the evidence base for their acceptability and effectiveness remained limited (Emmerton et al. 2003). The enthusiasm was real; the evidence was not yet in place to sustain it.

My PhD supervisors, Professor John P. Shaw and Associate Professor Lynne Emmerton, were among the researchers most committed to generating that evidence. They were designing and leading the Otago/Southland Comprehensive Pharmaceutical Care Asthma Project (Shaw et al. 1999), the first study in New Zealand to rigorously assess the impact of pharmaceutical care on the clinical and humanistic outcomes of patients with asthma. The project was conducted across community pharmacies in the Otago and Southland regions of the South Island, predominantly rural settings where pharmacist-patient relationships were enduring and trust was already woven into the fabric of daily life. Funded by the Health Funding Authority of New Zealand, with support from GlaxoWellcome New Zealand Limited, the study deployed a phase-in design across five pharmacies serving predominantly rural and established clientele, with patients acting as their own controls and receiving approximately monthly consultations with the pharmacist, including clinical and quality of life monitoring (Emmerton et al. 2003). The phase-in approach minimised disruption to pharmacists while maintaining the integrity of the before-and-after measurement.

During this period, our supervisory team was fortunate to be advised by Professor Charles Douglas Hepler himself, Distinguished Professor Emeritus at the University of Florida College of Pharmacy and co-architect, with Linda Strand, of the modern definition of pharmaceutical care. I had the privilege of dining with Professor Hepler in Dundee, a meeting that brought the human face of the intellectual framework we were working within into vivid personal relief, and confirmed that what we were attempting in rural New Zealand was precisely the kind of applied evidence-generation the founders of pharmaceutical care had envisioned as the profession's next obligation.

3.3 The PhD: Validation of Asthma Outcome Measures in the New Zealand Context

My role within the Otago/Southland project was specific, central and became the major pillar of my doctoral work. The thesis, titled Validation of Asthma Outcome Measures in the New Zealand Context (Kheir 2003), addressed a methodological question that had to be resolved before any of the clinical measurement could proceed: was the Asthma Quality of Life Questionnaire (AQLQ), the instrument of choice for measuring humanistic outcomes in asthma pharmaceutical care research, valid and responsive in the New Zealand patient population? This was not a trivial question. Patient-reported outcome measures developed in one cultural and linguistic context cannot be assumed to capture the same constructs with equivalent precision in another. The New Zealand population is multicultural, with Māori and Pacific communities whose illness experience, language and cultural frameworks may differ substantially from those of the populations in which the AQLQ was originally developed and validated. Establishing the instrument's fitness for purpose in this context was a prerequisite for any meaningful measurement, and it was a prerequisite that had not been met.

The process of cultural adaptation and validation involved systematic review of the AQLQ's items for cultural and linguistic relevance to the New Zealand context, consultation with clinicians and patients, and psychometric testing to establish that the instrument's measurement properties, including its reliability, validity and responsiveness to change, held in the New Zealand asthma population. It was painstaking work, and it was work that the published literature at the time largely overlooked: most pharmaceutical care outcome studies deployed existing instruments without examining their cross-cultural validity, a methodological shortcut that risks measuring nothing in particular with great precision.

In retrospect, this doctoral work was my true entry point into the science of patient-reported outcome measurement and validation, a field that would continue to shape my research agenda for the following two decades. The questions it raised, what does it mean for a questionnaire to be valid across cultures? How do we establish that what we are measuring in one population captures the same construct in another? How do we distinguish genuine clinical improvement from measurement artefact? The questions it raised, what does it mean for a questionnaire to be valid across cultures, how do we establish that what we are measuring in one population captures the same construct in another, how do we distinguish genuine clinical improvement from measurement artefact, these were questions I carried into every subsequent research programme, from the Arabic LMQ adaptation documented in Chap. 2 of this book to the treatment burden measurement work in Qatar.

3.4 The Study and Its Findings

The AQLQ, once validated for the New Zealand context, was deployed as the primary humanistic outcome measure across the Otago/Southland project. Adult asthma patients, 17 years of age and older, living in the Otago and Southland regions, were recruited and introduced to the pharmaceutical care service in phased cohorts, allowing them to act as their own controls and enabling before-and-after measurement within the same individuals (Kheir et al. 2001). The results were compelling: there was a significant improvement in asthma-related quality of life following the introduction of the service, as measured by the AQLQ, and pharmacists were able to identify, prevent or resolve more than 400 drug-related problems across the patient cohort (Kheir et al. 2001). The full demonstration project, reported by Emmerton et al. (2003), enrolled 100 patients across five pharmacies over 2 years, and found that on average 4.3 medication-related problems were identified per patient, two-thirds of them compliance-related. Clinical outcomes, including symptom control and inhaler technique, also improved.

What made these findings significant was not their magnitude in isolation but their context. This was New Zealand in the late 1990s, and pharmaceutical care was still a relatively new and contested philosophy of practice. The demonstration that trained community pharmacists, working in rural settings with established patient relationships and a structured service model, could generate measurable improvements in patients' quality of life and resolve hundreds of drug-related problems was not a foregone conclusion. It was evidence, produced with methodological care, for a proposition the profession needed to be able to defend.

Subsequent analysis of the AQLQ's psychometric performance in this setting, published in Kheir et al. (2008a), added an important layer of nuance. Three of the AQLQ's four domains, Activity Limitation, Symptoms, and Emotional Function, demonstrated adequate responsiveness to the pharmaceutical care intervention, confirming their utility as outcome measures in longitudinal pharmaceutical care studies. The fourth domain, Environmental Stimuli, showed weaker responsiveness, a finding with direct implications for researchers designing future studies: an instrument domain that does not detect clinically meaningful change is not merely uninformative; it is potentially misleading. The 2008 paper was, in this sense, as important for what it cautioned against as for what it confirmed.

The conceptual implications of all of this measurement work were drawn together in a paper co-authored with colleagues including Professor Foppe van Mil (Kheir et al. 2004), one of Europe's leading pharmaceutical care researchers, which argued that quality of life assessment is not merely a methodological tool in pharmaceutical care research but an ethical imperative. The shift in healthcare emphasis from disease and death to the management of illness had made it essential that healthcare providers assess the patient's experience as a legitimate outcome in its own right. Pharmaceutical care, with its explicit commitment to improving the patient's quality of life, had both the philosophical mandate and, through validated instruments like the AQLQ, the methodological means to do so. What remained was the professional will and the systemic infrastructure to make it routine.

3.5 What the Field Did With These Publications?

The citation record for this cluster of publications is both gratifying and instructive. Kheir et al. (2001) was included in the first systematic review and meta-analysis of pharmacist-delivered asthma self-management support services globally, conducted by Dokbua et al. (2018) and published in the Journal of Managed Care and Specialty Pharmacy. Of 12 studies selected for meta-analysis from Australia, Canada, Denmark, Germany, New Zealand, the United Kingdom and the United States, the New Zealand work was one of three studies measuring health-related quality of life as a primary outcome, and its inclusion in that pooled analysis gave the individual study findings a statistical weight they could not have had in isolation. The meta-analysis concluded that pharmacist-delivered asthma self-management support services significantly improved asthma control and quality of life across diverse healthcare contexts, a conclusion in which Kheir et al. (2001) played a meaningful part.

Emmerton et al. (2003) has had a particularly broad citation reach. It was cited in a study developing asthma pharmaceutical care models in Indonesia

(Widayati et al. 2018), in a hospital pharmacy-based pharmaceutical care services study in Sudan published in 2008, and in an Australian randomised trial of a targeted pharmacy asthma service (Serhal et al. 2021), which explicitly cited both the New Zealand demonstration project and the quality of life paper in framing its own rationale. In the Serhal et al. (2021) paper, the authors described how asthma is a chronic condition where steps toward minimising patient burden, enhancing emotional wellbeing and improving ability to participate in daily life are key, citing Kheir et al. (2001) and Kheir et al. (2004) as the foundational references for that framing. This is exactly the kind of citation that demonstrates intellectual rather than merely bibliographic inheritance: later researchers using earlier work to articulate not just a finding but a value.

Kheir et al. (2004) has been cited in systematic reviews of pharmaceutical care outcomes research as a conceptual reference point for why quality of life measurement belongs at the centre of pharmaceutical care evaluation (Mohammed et al. 2016), and in the development of new patient-reported outcome instruments for pharmaceutical care settings, including the PROMPT-QoL instrument, where the earlier paper's argument about targeting an outcome that matters was explicitly adopted as a design principle. A Brazilian study of pharmaceutical care interventions in elderly outpatients (de Lyra et al. 2007) cited Kheir et al. (2001) in framing its own outcome measurement approach, illustrating the reach of a study conducted in rural New Zealand pharmacies into the methodology of research in Ribeirao Preto. A 2022 pharmacist education efficacy study in Malaysia cited both Kheir et al. (2001) and Emmerton et al. (2003) when describing the evidence base for pharmacist interventions on asthma quality of life.

3.6 The Gap the Research Left Open

The call in Emmerton et al. (2003) for further research to integrate pharmaceutical care into daily pharmacy practice in New Zealand went substantially unanswered for more than a decade. The service demonstrated its clinical and humanistic value in a rigorously conducted demonstration project. It did not become embedded in routine New Zealand community pharmacy practice. The reasons are familiar from Chap. 1 of this book, and they are structural rather than evidential: the absence of a funded service model, no remuneration mechanism for pharmaceutical care services beyond the dispensing fee, no regulatory requirement for pharmacist-led chronic disease management, and no systematic postgraduate training infrastructure to sustain the competency the demonstration project had shown was achievable.

The AQLQ responsiveness finding (Kheir et al. 2008a) identified a specific psychometric gap that subsequent researchers in pharmaceutical care have not fully resolved. The Environmental Stimuli domain's weak responsiveness in a pharmaceutical care intervention context reflects a genuine construct problem: the items in that domain, which concern responses to environmental triggers for asthma, may not be amenable to change through a pharmacist-delivered service regardless of how well that service is delivered. Whether this domain should be retained, modified or omitted in pharmaceutical care outcome studies is a question the subsequent literature has discussed but not definitively answered.

There is also a reflexive gap worth naming. The PhD thesis that underpinned this cluster of publications made a rigorous case for the importance of cultural adaptation and validation before deployment of patient-reported outcome measures, grounded specifically in the New Zealand context. The subsequent career trajectory documented in this book involved deploying and adapting outcome measures in Qatar and the wider Middle East, where the same methodological principles applied. The Arabic LMQ translation and the work on medication-related burden in Qatar, described in Chap. 2, are the direct intellectual descendants of the Otago PhD work. The methodology travelled with the researcher.

3.7 From Research to Teaching

Looking back now, this chapter of my career was about far more than asthma or pharmacists or even New Zealand. It was where I learned to take measurement seriously, not as a technical exercise, but as a moral one. To measure a patient's quality of life is to ask them what their life is actually like. To validate an instrument across cultures is to insist that the question be asked in a way the patient can truly answer. That commitment to rigorous, patient-centred measurement was seeded in the hills of Otago, and it became a defining thread running through everything that followed.

It also, quite deliberately, found its way into my teaching. As my understanding of questionnaire development, cultural adaptation and validation deepened through research, I became increasingly convinced that these were not merely skills for the specialist researcher but essential competencies for any pharmacist practising in a world where patient-reported outcomes were becoming central to the evaluation of care. A conscious decision was made to bring this body of knowledge into the classroom, weaving the principles of instrument development, psychometric testing and cross-cultural adaptation and validation into the teaching of both undergraduate and postgraduate pharmacy students, in New Zealand, in Qatar, and subsequently at Waikato. The goal was not to produce measurement specialists, but to produce graduates who could use outcome measures intelligently and interrogate them critically, understanding what it truly means for a questionnaire to be valid, reliable and responsive to change in the populations it is meant to serve. Research, in this sense, had not simply informed the teaching. It had transformed it.

3.8 Research Agenda Note

The New Zealand research programme documented in this chapter points toward five open questions that represent the most important unfinished work arising from that early demonstration of pharmaceutical care.

First: why do rigorously demonstrated pharmaceutical care services fail to embed in routine practice, and what would a funded, sustainable service model have required in the New Zealand of the early 2000s? A retrospective implementation analysis of the Otago/Southland project and of comparable demonstration projects internationally, examining funding, regulation, workforce and professional politics, would convert an acknowledged disappointment into transferable implementation knowledge.

Second: should the Environmental Stimuli domain of the AQLQ be retained, modified or omitted in pharmaceutical care outcome studies? The responsiveness analysis in Kheir et al. (2008a) identified a genuine construct problem that the subsequent literature has discussed but not resolved. A dedicated psychometric study, testing the domain's responsiveness across multiple pharmaceutical care trials and patient populations, would settle a measurement question that continues to affect trial design.

Third: which remuneration and commissioning models sustain pharmacist-delivered asthma services beyond the life of a funded study? The Australian targeted asthma service evaluated by Serhal et al. (2021) offers a contemporary comparator to the New Zealand demonstration project. A comparative health system analysis of the two countries' trajectories would identify the policy conditions under which demonstrated value becomes routine provision.

Fourth: which patient-reported outcome measures are genuinely responsive to pharmaceutical care interventions? The systematic review evidence, including Mohammed et al. (2016), shows that many trials use instruments poorly matched to the mechanisms of pharmacist interventions. A systematic programme of responsiveness testing across candidate instruments, of the kind this chapter's doctoral work performed for the AQLQ, remains the unglamorous but foundational measurement work the field still needs.

Fifth: are the standard asthma quality of life instruments valid and responsive for Māori and Pacific patients? The doctoral research recognised that instruments developed elsewhere cannot be assumed to transfer across cultural and linguistic contexts, and the multicultural composition of the New Zealand patient population makes this a live equity question. Formal cultural validation studies, conducted in partnership with Māori and Pacific communities, would complete the validation agenda that the thesis opened.[1]

References

de Lyra DP, Kheir N, Abriata JP, da Rocha CE, Dos Santos CB, Pelá IR (2007) Impact of pharmaceutical care interventions in the identification and resolution of drug-related problems and on quality of life in a group of elderly outpatients in Ribeirão Preto (SP), Brazil. Ther Clin Risk Manag 3(6):989–998

[1]Publications by the author of this book are marked with an asterisk (*) in references.

Dokbua S, Dilokthornsakul P, Chaiyakunapruk N, Saini B, Krass I, Dhippayom T (2018) Effects of an asthma self-management support service provided by community pharmacists: a systematic review and meta-analysis. J Manag Care Spec Pharm 24(11):1184–1196

Emmerton L, Shaw J, Kheir N (2003) Asthma management by New Zealand pharmacists: a pharmaceutical care demonstration project. J Clin Pharm Ther 28(5):395–402*

Hepler CD, Strand LM (1990) Opportunities and responsibilities in pharmaceutical care. Am J Hosp Pharm 47(3):533–543

Kheir N, Emmerton L, Shaw JP (2001) Can pharmacists influence the health-related quality of life of patients with asthma? The New Zealand pharmaceutical care experience. Sultan Qaboos Univ Med J 3(2):70–75*

Kheir NM (2003) Validation of asthma outcome measures in the New Zealand context. PhD thesis, University of Otago, Dunedin*

Kheir NM, Emmerton L, Shaw JP (2008) Assessing the responsiveness of the Asthma Quality of Life Questionnaire with pharmaceutical care. Pharm World Sci 30(4):322–328*

Kheir NM, van Mil JW, Shaw JP, Sheridan JL (2004) Health-related quality of life measurement in pharmaceutical care: targeting an outcome that matters. Pharm World Sci 26(3):125–128*

Mohammed MA, Moles RJ, Chen TF (2016) Impact of pharmaceutical care interventions on health-related quality-of-life outcomes: a systematic review and meta-analysis. Ann Pharmacother 50(10):862–881

Serhal S, Saini B, Bosnic-Anticevich S, Krass I, Emmerton L, Bereznicki B et al (2021) A targeted approach to improve asthma control using community pharmacists. Front Pharmacol 12:798263

Shaw JP, Emmerton L, Kheir N, Smith N, Clareburt R, Barron P (1999) Otago/Southland Comprehensive Pharmaceutical Care Asthma Project (final report). School of Pharmacy, University of Otago, Dunedin*

Widayati A, Virginia DM, Setiawan CH et al (2018) Pharmacists' views on the development of asthma pharmaceutical care model in Indonesia: a needs analysis study. Res Soc Admin Pharm 14(12):1172–1179

Chapter 4
Does the Pharmacist Make a Difference? Evaluating Pharmaceutical Interventions and Living with Ambiguity

4.1 The Anchor Publication

This chapter is built around a single publication: the protocol paper for the Acute Coronary Syndrome randomised controlled trial, published in BMJ Open as Zidan et al. (2016). Unlike the other anchor publications in this book, it is a protocol rather than an outcomes paper, a design document that appeared in the peer-reviewed literature before the results it was built to generate. That position, at the start of an evidence-generation process rather than its conclusion, makes this chapter somewhat unusual in its structure. It requires an account not only of what the research asked and what it produced, but of what it means to publish a protocol, what the obligation incurred by doing so actually is, and how the evidence that followed, most notably the quasi-experimental study by El Hajj et al. (2023), completed the cycle the protocol had opened. Read together, Zidan et al. (2016) and El Hajj et al. (2023) constitute a full circle from research question to outcome evidence, and that circle is worth examining in detail.

4.2 The Question the Research Was Trying to Answer

Every serious research programme begins with a question that cannot be answered by what already exists in the literature. In the case of the ACS trial, the question was precise: does a structured pharmacist-delivered intervention at discharge and in the post-discharge period improve medication adherence and reduce hospitalisation in patients with acute coronary syndrome in Qatar? The question was precise because the problem it addressed was precise. Cardiovascular diseases had become the leading cause of morbidity and mortality in Qatar, with 16,736 ACS admissions recorded at Hamad Medical Corporation between 1991 and 2010 (Zidan et al. 2016). Despite the existence of well-established, evidence-based secondary prevention therapy,

N. Kheir, *Medicines, Patients, and the Gaps Between*,
https://doi.org/10.1007/978-981-92-5395-1_4

comprising aspirin, a beta-blocker, an angiotensin-converting enzyme inhibitor or angiotensin receptor blocker, and a statin, fewer than 80% of ACS patients in Qatar were using this quadruple combination after discharge (Zidan et al. 2016). The gap between recommended and actual secondary prevention was not a knowledge problem on the part of clinicians. It was an implementation problem, and one with a measurable human cost: non-adherence to secondary prevention medications after ACS is independently associated with increased risk of subsequent cardiac events, rehospitalisation and mortality (Horwitz et al. 1990).

The pharmacist's potential role in closing this gap was well theorised but, in the Gulf context, unevaluated. International literature had shown that pharmacist-delivered transitions of care interventions, structured medication reconciliation and counselling at hospital discharge combined with post-discharge follow-up, could improve secondary prevention adherence and reduce readmission rates in ACS and other cardiac patient populations (Lau et al. 2021). But the Gulf health system context differs from the Western settings in which most of that evidence was generated: the patient population in Qatar is predominantly expatriate, linguistically diverse, with variable health literacy and limited continuity of care between hospital and primary care settings. Whether findings from North American or European studies would translate to Heart Hospital in Doha was an empirical question, not one that could be answered by inference from elsewhere.

4.3 The Design and What It Established

The ACS trial was registered on ClinicalTrials.gov (NCT02648243) and designed as a three-arm randomised controlled trial. The three arms compared: standard care alone; a pharmacist-delivered intervention consisting of medication reconciliation and counselling at discharge and a combined intervention comprising the discharge component plus tailored pharmacist-led follow-up at 3, 6, and 12 months post-discharge. The primary outcomes were hospital readmissions, emergency department visits, and all-cause mortality at 3, 6, and 12 months. Secondary outcomes included patient adherence to secondary prevention medications, patient satisfaction with pharmacy services and reduction in treatment burden (Zidan et al. 2016).

Publishing the protocol in BMJ Open was a deliberate act of scientific transparency, and it served several functions simultaneously. It established the trial's existence, design and pre-specified hypotheses in the peer-reviewed literature before any results were available, making the study accountable to its stated design in a way that unpublished trials cannot be. It created a citable reference point for other researchers in the region working on pharmacist-delivered cardiac care. It demonstrated that the Gulf pharmacy research community was capable of designing and registering rigorous clinical trials, at a time when the region was substantially underrepresented in the international clinical pharmacy literature. And it signalled to the global cardiovascular pharmacist community that Qatar was generating its own evidence base rather than simply importing and applying evidence produced elsewhere.

This matters because it represents a significant step in the maturation of a research programme. The surveys and observational studies that characterised much of the early Middle Eastern pharmacy research literature, including the work described in Chaps. 1 and 2 of this book, were necessary first steps. But surveys describe what exists; trials test what could be different. The ACS protocol represented a transition from description to intervention, from asking what is happening to asking what changes when we do something differently. That is a qualitatively different kind of research enterprise, and it requires a different kind of institutional support, including research governance infrastructure, ethics committee processes, clinical trial registration and the ability to sustain patient follow-up over 12 months in a health system where many patients may relocate, change employers or lose access to the same clinical team.

4.4 What the Trial Found: The El Hajj et al. (2023) Study

The full outcomes of the RCT as registered have not been published as a single completed trial paper at the time of writing. What has been published, and what represents the most direct evidence arising from the same institutional context, is the quasi-experimental study by El Hajj et al. (2023), conducted at Heart Hospital, Hamad Medical Corporation in Qatar, and explicitly citing Zidan et al. (2016) as its direct intellectual precursor. That study compared outcomes in 191 post-ACS patients who received a structured pharmacist-delivered intervention with 191 matched controls who received standard care. The primary outcomes were all-cause hospitalisation and cardiac-related hospital readmission at 6 months post-discharge.

The results were clinically meaningful: all-cause hospitalisation was significantly lower in the intervention group than in the control group, and cardiac-related readmissions were significantly reduced. The intervention consisted of medication reconciliation at discharge, patient education on secondary prevention medications and cardiovascular risk reduction, and follow-up telephone counselling at 1 and 3 months post-discharge. These are not exotic or expensive components. They are structured, trained, pharmacist-delivered services that can be operationalised within existing hospital pharmacy infrastructure, given adequate time, training and institutional mandate (El Hajj et al. 2023).

This result needs to be read in the context of the broader international evidence on pharmacist-led ACS interventions. The Canadian PRIMA-ACS study found that pharmacist-delivered discharge counselling alone was not associated with significantly better adherence at 1 year, and its authors observed that in the systematic review evidence available at the time, only a minority of studies showed improved adherence, typically those whose interventions extended beyond the hospital setting into post-discharge follow-up (Neville et al. 2021). A matched cohort study from Australia, published in 2023, found that a telehealth cardiology pharmacist clinic significantly improved adherence to secondary prevention medications at 12 months post-ACS compared with standard care (Livori et al. 2023). A randomised controlled trial from Vietnam, published in 2018, found significantly higher adherence at 1 and 3 months post-discharge in patients who received a pharmacist-delivered intervention compared with controls (Nguyen et al. 2018). The Qatar evidence, taken together with these international findings, supports a consistent directional conclusion: structured pharmacist involvement in the post-ACS transition of care improves both adherence and clinical outcomes, but only when the intervention is sufficiently intensive and extends beyond the hospital walls into the period when patients are managing their regimens at home.

4.5 What the Field Did with the Protocol?

The ACS trial protocol (Zidan et al. 2016) has been cited in the international literature in several distinct ways, each reflecting a different use of a protocol publication. It was cited in a systematic review of pharmacist-involved care for patients with heart failure and ACS by Lau et al. (2021), which identified it as one of the studies in the Gulf setting contributing to the evidence base for pharmacist-led cardiac care. It was cited in Pharmacy Times clinical guidance on acute coronary syndrome management, where the protocol was referenced to support the argument that pharmacists have a demonstrable role in post-ACS secondary prevention support. And it was cited in the El Hajj et al. (2023) quasi-experimental study as the direct methodological and intellectual ancestor of that subsequent work, establishing an explicit continuity between the question the protocol asked and the evidence the outcomes study provided.

This last citation is, in some respects, the most important. The protocol-to-outcomes citation trail is the mechanism by which a published protocol fulfils its purpose: the design is established in the record, subsequent researchers build on or test it, and the field accumulates evidence in an organised rather than ad hoc fashion. The fact that the same institution, Heart Hospital in Qatar, generated both the protocol and the subsequent quasi-experimental outcomes study illustrates how a published research design can anchor a sustained programme of clinical inquiry rather than existing as a stand-alone publication.

4.6 The Ambiguity the Evidence Leaves Behind

Acknowledging what the research achieved requires equal honesty about what it did not resolve. The ambiguity embedded in the pharmacist-impact literature is real, persistent and worth confronting rather than papering over with selectively cited positive findings. The PRIMA-ACS report noted that only four of twelve studies in the systematic review evidence it drew upon showed improved adherence in the ACS patient population and those were characterised by small sample sizes and interventions that extended beyond the hospital setting (Neville et al. 2021). The evidence that pharmacist-delivered discharge counselling alone, without post-discharge follow-up, produces durable improvements in adherence is weak. The evidence that more intensive, extended interventions produce meaningful outcomes is stronger but still heterogeneous.

What this ambiguity means, practically, is that the answer to the question this chapter poses:, i.e "*does the pharmacist make a difference?*" cannot be given as a simple yes. The more accurate and more useful answer is: "*yes, under specifiable conditions*". When the intervention is structured and delivered by a trained pharmacist, when it extends from the hospital into the post-discharge period, when the patient population has been identified through clear inclusion criteria, and when the outcome measurement is sufficiently sensitive to detect the relevant changes over an adequate time horizon, the evidence consistently points toward a meaningful pharmacist contribution to post-ACS secondary prevention. But these conditions are not easily satisfied. They require sustained institutional investment in pharmacist training, dedicated clinical time for patient education and post-discharge follow-up, and a formally recognised professional mandate within the cardiac care team, conditions that are rarely guaranteed by the completion of a single study, however, well designed. Whether they have been systematically established and maintained in the Qatar hospital setting beyond the life of the research programme is a question the published literature cannot answer, and one that institutional leaders have yet to address publicly.

4.7 The Deeper Question: Proof of Concept Versus Standard of Care

There is a tension embedded in the entire pharmacist-impact literature that the ACS work at Heart Hospital illustrates particularly clearly. Research studies demonstrate that pharmacist-delivered interventions can produce positive outcomes under controlled conditions. The healthcare systems in which those studies are conducted then face the question of whether to institutionalise the intervention as a standard of care, which requires sustained funding, staffing and professional mandate, rather than simply acknowledging that a proof of concept has been established.

In Qatar, as in most of the Gulf, the gap between proof of concept and standard of care remains wide. The El Hajj et al. (2023) study demonstrated that a structured post-ACS pharmacist intervention reduced readmissions at a specific hospital during a specific study period. Whether that intervention has been integrated into the routine discharge and post-discharge care of ACS patients at Heart Hospital, whether it is reliably delivered to every eligible patient regardless of research status, whether pharmacists have the protected time and clinical mandate to sustain it at scale, are questions that the published literature cannot answer and that institutional leaders have not yet answered publicly. The evidence exists. The infrastructure to act on it consistently does not yet exist in the same measure. That gap is not unique to Qatar; it is the defining implementation challenge of clinical pharmacy globally. But naming it honestly, in a book that reflects on a research programme rather than simply celebrating it, is part of the scholarly obligation this chapter owes its reader.

4.8 Research Agenda Note

The ACS research programme documented in this chapter points toward five open questions that represent the most important unfinished work on pharmacist-delivered cardiovascular interventions in the region.

First: how can structured post-ACS pharmacist involvement be sustained, scaled and embedded as the default in routine care rather than delivered as a study condition? The efficacy question has been answered in the directionally consistent international evidence this chapter reviews. The implementation science questions, concerning barriers to routine delivery, workforce requirements and the systems changes that make the intervention ordinary, remain almost entirely open in the Gulf context.

Second: what is the cost-effectiveness of extended post-discharge pharmacist interventions after ACS? Health system planners cannot invest in expanded pharmacist roles on clinical evidence alone. A formal economic evaluation alongside the next intervention study, capturing readmission costs averted against intervention delivery costs, is the single missing piece of evidence most likely to change commissioning decisions.

Third: what intervention intensity and duration are actually necessary? The pattern across the evidence reviewed in this chapter, in which discharge counselling alone shows little effect while interventions extending into the post-discharge period show benefit, implies a dose-response relationship that no study has tested directly. A trial comparing discharge-only, short extended and long extended pharmacist follow-up would define the minimum effective dose of post-ACS pharmaceutical care.

Fourth: do culturally and linguistically adapted post-ACS interventions produce more equitable outcomes in heterogeneous patient populations? The Heart Hospital catchment is linguistically diverse in ways the original protocol did not fully accommodate. Testing structured counselling delivered in patients' first languages against standard delivery, with adherence and readmission stratified by language group, would address an equity gap that current protocols quietly assume away.

Fifth: which components of the multicomponent intervention drive its effect? Medication reconciliation, discharge counselling and follow-up contact travel together in most protocols, including Zidan et al. (2016). Factorial designs or rigorous process evaluations that decompose the intervention would tell the field what to protect when resources force simplification.

4.9 What Remains?

The ACS research programme at Heart Hospital points toward an agenda that is clear in its direction if not yet in its completion. The next generation of research in this space needs to move from demonstrating that pharmacist-delivered post-ACS interventions work under study conditions to testing how they can be sustained, scaled and embedded in routine care. That requires implementation science rather than efficacy science: studies that examine the barriers to routine delivery, the workforce and systems changes needed to make structured post-ACS pharmacist involvement the default rather than the exception, and the cost-effectiveness evidence that would allow health system planners to invest in expanded pharmacist roles with confidence.

It also requires a more systematic engagement with patient diversity. The ACS patient population at Heart Hospital in Qatar is linguistically and culturally heterogeneous in ways that most intervention protocols, including the one documented in Zidan et al. (2016), did not fully account for. A patient counselled in English who speaks Urdu or Tagalog as a first language is not receiving equivalent care to a patient counselled in their native tongue, regardless of how structured and well trained the pharmacist delivering that counselling may be. Culturally and linguistically adapted post-ACS pharmacist interventions, tested in the specific population of Heart Hospital's catchment, represent a research gap that both the equity agenda and the effectiveness agenda demand be filled.[1]

References

El Hajj MS, Kaddoura R, Abu Yousef SEA, Orabi B, Awaisu A, AlYafei S, Shami R, Mahfoud ZR (2023) Effectiveness of a structured pharmacist-delivered intervention for patients post-acute coronary syndromes on all-cause hospitalizations and cardiac-related hospital readmissions: a prospective quasi-experimental study. Int J Clin Pharm 45(3):630–640

Horwitz RI, Viscoli CM, Berkman L, Donaldson RM, Horwitz SM, Murray CJ, Ransohoff DF, Sindelar J (1990) Treatment adherence and risk of death after a myocardial infarction. Lancet 336(8714):542–545

Lau WCY et al (2021) Pharmacist-involved care for patients with heart failure and acute coronary syndrome: a systematic review with qualitative and quantitative meta-analysis. Br J Clin Pharmacol 87(10):3761–3782

Livori AC, Pol D, Levkovich B, Oqueli E (2023) Optimising adherence to secondary prevention medications following acute coronary syndrome utilising telehealth cardiology pharmacist clinics: a matched cohort study. Int J Clin Pharm 45(3):722–730

Neville HL, Mann K, Killen J, Callaghan M (2021) Pharmacist intervention to improve medication adherence in patients with acute coronary syndrome: the PRIMA-ACS study. Can J Hosp Pharm 74(4):350–360

Nguyen T, Nguyen TH, Nguyen PT, Tran HT, Nguyen NV, Nguyen HQ, Ha BN, Pham TT, Taxis K (2018) Pharmacist-led intervention to enhance medication adherence in patients with acute coronary syndrome in Vietnam: a randomized controlled trial. Front Pharmacol 9:656

Zidan A, Awaisu A, Kheir N, Mahfoud Z, Kaddoura R, AlYafei S, El Hajj MS (2016) Impact of a pharmacist-delivered discharge and follow-up intervention for patients with acute coronary syndromes in Qatar: a study protocol for a randomised controlled trial. BMJ Open 6(11):e012141*

[1]Publications by the author of this book are marked with an asterisk (*) in references.

Chapter 5
Counselling, Communication and the Gap at the Counter

5.1 The Anchor Publication

This chapter is built around Paravattil et al. (2017), published in the International Journal of Clinical Pharmacy, which used trained actors to visit 136 private community pharmacies across Qatar and present pharmacists with standardised clinical scenarios for two of the most commonly dispensed medication classes in the country: a salbutamol inhaler for asthma and glimepiride for diabetes. Pharmacists were unaware that they were being assessed. What the simulated patients recorded was not what pharmacists said they did, or what they intended to do, or what they reported doing in a survey conducted after the fact. It was what they actually did in a real clinical encounter, under real conditions, with a real person standing at the counter asking for help. The gap between those two things, what pharmacists say and what pharmacists do, is where the most important and most uncomfortable evidence in pharmacy practice research tends to live.

5.2 Why the Simulated Patient Method Matters?

The simulated patient methodology has a specific and irreplaceable function in pharmacy practice research. Unlike surveys, which capture self-reported attitudes and behaviours subject to social desirability bias, or observations, which alter behaviour through the awareness of being watched, the simulated patient method captures practice as it actually occurs in the moment of the encounter. The pharmacist who knows they are being observed tends to perform better than they would otherwise; the pharmacist who does not know is simply doing their job. This distinction is not merely methodological. It is the difference between knowing what pharmacists aspire to do and knowing what patients actually receive.

N. Kheir, *Medicines, Patients, and the Gaps Between*,
https://doi.org/10.1007/978-981-92-5395-1_5

The method is not without limitations, and these deserve direct acknowledgement. A simulated patient can only present one type of encounter; they cannot replicate the full complexity of a patient with multiple conditions, multiple medications and a history of interaction with the same pharmacist over years. The scenarios must be scripted and standardised, which means they capture what the pharmacist does when the clinical context is clear and the patient is cooperative, not necessarily what happens when the consultation is time-pressured, ambiguous, or complicated by language barriers. And simulated patients, however, well trained, are actors performing illness rather than people living it, which may produce slightly different responses from pharmacists attuned to non-verbal or emotional cues. These limitations are real, but they do not undermine the method's fundamental contribution: it produces the most ecologically valid picture of routine pharmacy practice currently available to researchers.

The Qatar study was designed to examine not only the quality of counselling provided but also the factors that predicted it. One hundred and thirty-six community pharmacies were visited by trained simulated patients presenting four scenarios: a new prescription for salbutamol, a salbutamol refill, a new prescription for glimepiride and a glimepiride refill. A structured assessment form captured the counselling provided across multiple domains, including information on the medication's name, purpose, dosing, administration technique, side effects and follow-up. After each simulated visit, the pharmacist completed a questionnaire that allowed the researchers to examine the relationship between counselling quality and patient characteristics, pharmacist characteristics and pharmacy characteristics (Paravattil et al. 2017).

5.3 What the Study Found: A Portrait of Routine Practice

Unfortunately, the findings of Paravattil et al. (2017) were not shocking to anyone who had spent time observing community pharmacy practice in numerous regions, worldwide. They were, however, precise, and precision in a field accustomed to vague impressions and self-reported optimism carries its own discomfort. The majority of pharmacists provided information about the medication's name. Fewer provided information about its purpose. Fewer still provided information about dosing, administration or side effects. Disease management, the kind of patient-centred conversation that pharmaceutical care requires, in which the pharmacist explores the patient's understanding of their condition, assesses their adherence to existing therapy, identifies potential drug-related problems, and tailors their advice to the individual's circumstances, was largely absent.

The asthma scenario produced particularly striking results. Only two pharmacists in the entire study, representing 6.2% of those presenting the salbutamol scenario, correctly demonstrated all required steps of inhaler technique (Paravattil et al. 2017). Inhaler technique is not a peripheral aspect of asthma care. It is a fundamental determinant of whether the medication reaches the airways at all. A patient who is prescribed a salbutamol inhaler and sent home without instruction on how to use it is not receiving treatment in any clinically meaningful sense; they are receiving a device they do not know how to operate. That 93.8% of pharmacists in this study failed to provide complete instruction on inhaler technique is not a data point about individual pharmacist inadequacy. It is a finding about the structural conditions of community pharmacy practice in Qatar at a specific point in time.

The diabetes scenario was equally revealing. More than 60% of pharmacists, when asked about glimepiride therapy by a patient presenting for a refill, referred the patient to the physician as their primary response. In isolation, this might appear to reflect appropriate professional caution, recognising the limits of the pharmacist's role and directing patients toward the prescriber for clinical decisions. But in context, it reflects something more troubling: a professional identity that had not yet accommodated the expectation that the pharmacist would directly counsel the patient about their diabetes medication, its mechanism, its side effects, its administration and its management in everyday life. The pharmacist was not declining to perform a function they recognised as theirs. They were declining to perform a function they had not been given reason to regard as theirs.

The finding that male patients received significantly better counselling than female patients was among the most uncomfortable in the dataset (Paravattil et al. 2017). Qatar's community pharmacy workforce at the time of the study was predominantly male, and the interaction between pharmacist gender, patient gender and cultural norms around same-gender professional interaction appears to have produced a systematic inequity in the counselling female patients received. This is not a finding that the study was designed to investigate in depth, and the data do not permit conclusions about the mechanism. But the finding is real, and its implications for equity of access to pharmaceutical care in a multicultural, gender-stratified healthcare environment are significant and remain inadequately addressed in the regional literature.

One structural predictor of counselling quality deserves particular attention. The absence of a private counselling area, identifiable in the post-visit pharmacist questionnaire as a characteristic of some pharmacies, was associated with lower counselling scores. This is the most direct empirical confirmation in the Qatar literature of what the structural analysis in Chapters One and Six of this book argues at length: the conditions of the physical environment shape clinical behaviour as powerfully as any training programme. A pharmacist who cannot offer a patient a private space for a clinical conversation is not simply less comfortable; they are structurally constrained from providing a standard of care that pharmaceutical care requires.

5.4 What the Field Did with This Publication?

Paravattil et al. (2017) entered a literature that was already using the simulated patient method across the MENA region but had produced relatively few studies that combined multiple scenarios, multiple pharmacy characteristics, and a randomised visit design in a single study. Its citation record reflects both the breadth of the methodology and the specificity of its findings.

The paper was cited in the CPD needs assessment study conducted in Qatar by Al-Sulaiti et al. (2021), which used the counselling gap it documented as direct justification for the design and content of a structured continuing professional development programme. The Al-Sulaiti et al. (2021) study found that pharmaceutical care process and drug information skills were the most identified topics for inclusion in CPD programmes, precisely consistent with the deficiencies Paravattil et al. (2017) had quantified. This is a clean example of the full-circle architecture this book describes: research identifies the gap, the gap informs the educational response, the educational response cites the research as its justification.

The paper was included in a systematic review of simulated patient methodology in the MENA region published in 2022, which identified it as one of the methodologically stronger regional studies, noting its randomised visit design and its examination of pharmacist, patient, and pharmacy characteristics as predictors of counselling quality. It was cited in a UAE simulated patient study of asthma pharmacist practice (Hasan et al. 2021), in an Ethiopian multi-centre study of community pharmacists' roles in asthma education published in 2020, in a Brazilian pharmacist training evaluation study published in 2020, in a Canadian men's mental health pharmacy programme evaluation published in 2018, and in a systematic review of simulated patient methodology in childhood diarrhoea management published in 2023. It was cited as recently as 2025 in a study of asthma patient education and counselling in community pharmacies in Kurdistan Region, Iraq (Yassen et al. 2025).

This citation pattern is geographically striking. A study of community pharmacy counselling in Qatar has been cited in research conducted in Canada, Brazil, Ethiopia, Iraq, the UAE and Iran. The research did not stay in the Gulf. It became part of an international methodological and substantive conversation about what community pharmacists do when patients ask for help with chronic disease management, and about what the simulated patient method reveals that surveys cannot. That conversation is still ongoing.

5.5 The Structural Explanation: Why Training Alone Is Insufficient?

The most common institutional response to the findings of a simulated patient counselling study is to call for more training. If pharmacists are providing incomplete inhaler technique demonstrations, the solution appears obvious: train them better. If they are failing to discuss side effects, add side effect counselling to the continuing professional development programme. This response is not wrong, but it is radically insufficient, and the pharmacy practice literature has been demonstrating its insufficiency for long enough that the field should, by now, be drawing different conclusions.

The pharmacists documented in Paravattil et al. (2017) were not, in the main, untrained. The majority had completed undergraduate pharmacy programmes that included communication skills training, pharmaceutical care principles, and clinical pharmacy content. Qatar University's College of Pharmacy, which was producing graduates at the time the study was conducted, offered a curriculum with demonstrably high standards for pharmaceutical care education, as documented by Awaisu et al. (2018) and described in Chap. 1 of this book. The problem was not that pharmacists did not know how to counsel patients. The problem was that the environment in which they worked did not create the conditions, the time, the space, or the professional standing that would make counselling the default rather than the exception.

A pharmacist processing over 40 prescription transactions in a shift has approximately 90 seconds of counseling per patient. A pharmacist operating from a counter open to a busy retail environment has no confidential space in which to discuss a patient's blood glucose control or their difficulty remembering to take a twice-daily medication. A pharmacist whose employer measures performance in terms of prescription throughput, not patient outcomes, has no incentive structure that rewards the time spent on a counselling conversation. These are not individual failures. They are systemic conditions, and the simulated patient study documented their consequences with quantitative precision.

The finding about private counselling areas is the most direct evidence in the Paravattil et al. (2017) data that structural conditions predict clinical behaviour. But it is the tip of a much larger iceberg. The full structural picture includes the physical layout of the pharmacy, the staffing levels, the workload per shift, the legal framework that defines the pharmacist's professional obligations and liabilities, the remuneration system that determines what is financially rational to spend time on, and the professional culture that shapes what pharmacists believe they are expected to provide. No training programme, however, sophisticated, can compensate for a structural environment that makes counselling impractical, unrewarded and professionally unrecognised.

5.6 The Gap the Research Left Open

Paravattil et al. (2017) documented what community pharmacists in Qatar were doing in 2014 and 2015, the years in which the data were collected. What it could not do was explain in sufficient depth why they were doing it or test what would happen if the structural conditions it identified as barriers were changed. The study identified the absence of private counselling areas as a predictor of lower counselling quality, but it did not test whether providing those areas would improve practice. It identified pharmacist characteristics such as academic qualification as associated with counselling quality, but it did not examine the specific content of those qualifications or the quality of the clinical training that had accompanied them. It identified patient gender as a predictor of counselling quality but did not investigate the mechanisms or explore the perspectives of the pharmacists whose behaviour produced the inequity.

These are not criticisms of the study's design, which was appropriate for its stated aims. They are an honest account of what a cross-sectional simulated patient study can and cannot tell us. The research contributed a precisely documented baseline. It did not, and could not, generate the implementation evidence that would allow pharmacy managers, professional bodies, and health system planners to know which specific structural interventions would produce the most significant improvements in counselling practice. That implementation evidence, the result of rigorously designed studies that test specific changes to the pharmacy environment and measure their effect on what pharmacists actually do, remains largely absent from the Qatar literature and from the MENA region more broadly.

There is also a temporal gap worth acknowledging. The data in Paravattil et al. (2017) were collected more than a decade ago. Community pharmacy in Qatar has changed since then, at least in some respects: the CPD programme that Al-Sulaiti et al. (2021) documented was developed partly in response to the evidence this study provided, and Qatar's National Health Strategy has continued to articulate ambitions for expanded pharmacist roles in primary care. Whether those changes have produced measurable improvements in the quality of counselling that patients actually receive at the counter is a question that a follow-up simulated patient study in the same setting, with the same methodology, would be uniquely well positioned to answer. That study has not been conducted, at least at the time of writing.

5.7 Research Agenda Note

The counselling research documented in this chapter points toward five open questions that represent the most important unfinished work on the quality of patient counselling at the community pharmacy counter.

First: has counselling practice in Qatar's community pharmacies changed since the 2014 and 2015 data documented in Paravattil et al. (2017)? A repeat simulated patient study in the same setting, using the same methodology and scenarios, is uniquely well positioned to answer this, and it has not been done. Given the CPD programmes and policy ambitions that the original study helped justify, the follow-up study is also a test of whether those responses achieved anything measurable at the counter.

Second: does changing the structural conditions the original study identified actually improve counselling quality? The study found that the absence of private counselling areas predicted poorer counselling, but prediction is not proof of remedy. Quasi-experimental studies in which specific structural changes, private consultation spaces, adjusted staffing levels or altered remuneration are introduced and counselling quality is measured before and after would generate the implementation evidence that managers and regulators currently lack.

Third: what mechanisms produce the patient-gender inequity in counselling quality that the study documented? The finding was reported; the explanation was not investigated. Qualitative research with practising pharmacists, exploring the social norms, assumptions, and interactional dynamics that shape counselling encounters with male and female patients, is the necessary next step before any corrective training can be designed with confidence.

Fourth: which elements of a pharmacist's education and training actually predict counselling quality? Academic qualification was associated with better counselling, but a credential is a proxy not a mechanism. Research that examines the content of qualifications, particularly the presence and quality of supervised clinical communication training, would identify what to strengthen in the curricula and CPD programmes that feed the community pharmacy workforce.

Fifth: what counselling do patients themselves want, absorb and act upon? The simulated patient method measures what pharmacists deliver against professional standards; it cannot measure what real patients value or use. Studies linking observed counselling quality to patient comprehension, adherence and outcomes would shift the field's endpoint from checklist completeness to patient benefit, which is where this book has argued the endpoint always belonged.

5.8 What Remains?

The counselling gap documented in Paravattil et al. (2017) is a specific instance of a general problem that this book has returned to in different forms across multiple chapters: the distance between the pharmaceutical care that the profession articulates as its mission and the pharmaceutical care that patients actually receive. In Chap. 1, that distance was described as a structural decoupling between education and practice. In Chap. 2, it was described as the gap between measuring treatment burden and intervening on it. In Chap. 5, it is the gap between a trained pharmacist standing behind a counter and a patient leaving that counter without the counselling that would have made their medication safer, more effective, and more likely to be taken. Chapters 6 and 7 examine the same structural failure from the perspectives of pharmacy education and research capacity respectively, each arriving at a version of the same conclusion: that the community pharmacy, as currently constituted across most of the region, is an environment that resists the improvements that education, research and professional aspiration are simultaneously trying to deliver.

Closing that gap requires a different kind of research agenda from the one that produced Paravattil et al. (2017). It requires implementation studies that test specific changes to the pharmacy environment, the staffing model, the remuneration structure and the professional expectation framework, and measure their effect on what pharmacists do. It requires studies that distinguish between pharmacists who counsel poorly because they do not know how and pharmacists who counsel poorly because the conditions of their practice make counselling impractical, because the interventions needed to address those two groups are entirely different. And it requires sustained advocacy, from the research community to policy makers and pharmacy owners, that translates the evidence of the counselling gap into the systemic changes that training programmes alone will never achieve.[1]

[1]Publications by the author of this book are marked with an asterisk (*) in references.

References

Al-Sulaiti F, Fares H, Awaisu A, Kheir N (2021) Continuing professional development needs of community pharmacists in Qatar: a mixed-methods approach. Int Q Community Health Educ 41(3):285–292*

Awaisu A, Katoue MG, Al-Taweel D, Bacha R, El-Gargawi A, Kheir N (2018) Self-reported attitudes and perceived preparedness to provide pharmaceutical care among final year pharmacy students in Qatar and Kuwait. Pharm Educ 18(1):284–291*

Hasan S, Al Oum L, Hassan NA (2021) A simulated patient study to evaluate community pharmacist assessment, management and advice giving to patients with asthma. J Pharm Policy Pract 14. https://doi.org/10.1186/s40545-020-00294-4

Paravattil B, Kheir N, Yousif A (2017) Utilization of simulated patients to assess diabetes and asthma counseling practices among community pharmacists in Qatar. Int J Clin Pharm 39(4):759–768*

Yassen AO, Shlaymoon AS, Ghanim Salem N, Shakir SA (2025) Asthma patient education and counselling in community pharmacies in Kurdistan Region, Erbil, Iraq: a cross-sectional study. Int Pharm Acta 8(1):e7

Chapter 6
Staying Current: Continuing Professional Development and the Gap Between Training and Practice

6.1 The Problem CPD Is Trying to Solve

Continuing professional development (CPD) exists because the knowledge that graduates acquire at school has a half-life. Drug formularies change. Guidelines are revised. New roles emerge that undergraduate programmes did not anticipate. Diseases that were once managed in hospital settings migrate into community care. Patients arrive with comorbidities, polypharmacy regimens and cultural contexts that no single training programme can fully prepare a pharmacist to navigate. The pharmacist who graduated competently a decade ago may, without sustained effort, find themselves practising with a knowledge base that is no longer adequate to the demands placed upon it.

This is not a pharmacy-specific problem. Every health profession confronts it, and every health profession has developed some version of an answer: continuing education requirements, postgraduate certificates, clinical updates, professional development programmes, reflective practice frameworks, peer review. The diversity of these responses reflects the genuine difficulty of the underlying challenge: how do you keep a distributed, heterogeneous workforce current in a rapidly evolving field, at acceptable cost, with mechanisms that actually change what practitioners do rather than simply generating evidence that they attended something?

In Qatar, this challenge arrived with particular urgency during the first decade of this century. The pharmacy profession there was young, rapidly expanding and overwhelmingly expatriate in composition. Pharmacists trained in Egypt, India, Jordan and Sudan practised alongside fresh graduates of Qatar University's new College of Pharmacy, which had opened in 2007 with a curriculum built around pharmaceutical care principles that many practising pharmacists had never encountered in their own training. The gap between what contemporary pharmacy education aspired to produce and what the practising workforce could currently deliver was not a gap that goodwill alone could close. It required structured, evidence-based, carefully designed continuing

N. Kheir, *Medicines, Patients, and the Gaps Between*,
https://doi.org/10.1007/978-981-92-5395-1_6

professional development, and it required an honest assessment of whether what CPD delivered was actually changing practice.

Several publications from our research group addressed these questions across a span of 15 years, and what they reveal, taken together, is a story with more complications than the CPD literature typically acknowledges. It is a story about the limits of self-report as a basis for programme design, about the stubbornly persistent gap between knowledge acquisition and behaviour change, and about the structural conditions in practice environments that determine whether training, however, well designed, actually translates into different care.

6.2 The JCEHP Study: Can Pharmacists Tell You What They Need?

The first major question our research group addressed was methodological: is self-assessment of CPD needs a reliable basis for programme design? The intuitive answer is that it should be. Practising pharmacists know what they do not know, or at least they should. They encounter knowledge gaps in their daily practice. They know which patient questions they cannot answer confidently, which clinical scenarios make them uncomfortable, which areas of pharmacotherapy have advanced beyond their current understanding. A needs assessment that asks pharmacists directly about their training requirements ought, in principle, to yield a useable picture of the profession's collective CPD needs.

The reality, as Kheir, Al-Ismail, and Al-Nakeeb (2017) found in a cross-sectional study conducted in Qatar and published in the Journal of Continuing Education in the Health Professions, is considerably more complicated. The study used a triangulation approach, a strategy borrowed from qualitative research methodology, to compare three simultaneous assessments of pharmacist competence: pharmacists' own self-assessments, assessments by pharmacy students who had completed structured experiential training rotations in multiple pharmacy settings, and assessments by pharmacy managers and academics. The questionnaire drew on the National Association of Pharmacy Regulatory Authorities (NAPRA) professional competency framework, which structured the assessment across seven domains including patient care, professional collaboration, drug information, communication and management.

The findings were uncomfortable. Across virtually every competency domain assessed, pharmacists rated their own competence significantly higher than either students or managers rated it. The self-assessed competency level was consistently higher than what observers reported, with statistically significant differences between pharmacist self-assessments and both student and manager observations ($p < 0.001$ for most domains). Sixty-five percent of pharmacists described themselves as fully or reasonably satisfied with their competency level. By contrast, only 21% of observing students and 14% of managers expressed equivalent satisfaction with what they had observed. The pattern was not marginal. It was systemic and substantial.

This is the Dunning–Kruger problem in a pharmacy practice setting: the phenomenon, described in the psychological literature, in which people with limited competence in a domain tend to overestimate their own performance because the same knowledge gaps that limit their competence also limit their ability to recognise that limitation. Pharmacists who assessed themselves as reasonably competent in pharmaceutical care delivery may simply have had an insufficiently demanding concept of what pharmaceutical care delivery requires, a concept shaped by years of practising in an environment where a narrower, more product-focused conception of the pharmacist's role was the norm.

There were also differences in what pharmacists and observers identified as training priorities. Pharmacists placed relatively less emphasis than students and managers on needs in health promotion, pharmacy practice research and pharmacy management, areas that observers regarded as significantly underdeveloped. Pharmacists, by contrast, gravitated toward fact-intensive topics: pharmacotherapy of disease states, drug information, dispensing skills. This pattern is consistent with what the needs assessment literature describes as the distinction between wants, needs and demands: pharmacists wanted training in areas they already partially understood and found professionally comfortable, while observers identified needs in areas that were less visible to pharmacists precisely because they were underdeveloped.

What did this mean for CPD programme design? The triangulation approach, despite its conceptual appeal, left the research team with a genuine dilemma that the paper named honestly. If pharmacists' self-assessments are unreliable, designing programmes based on them risks addressing the wrong things. But designing programmes based entirely on what students and managers observed, overriding pharmacists' own professional judgement about what they need, raises a different problem: it is paternalistic, potentially counterproductive to engagement and may not improve uptake or motivation. The paper advocated for rubric-based self-assessment tools and reflection-in-action strategies as potential bridges between self-report and external observation, but acknowledged that the practical value of these approaches in making CPD planning decisions remained unclear. The honest conclusion was that source triangulation, while intellectually interesting, did not resolve the core difficulty: the profession's tools for identifying its own learning needs may be systematically biased in ways that the profession is poorly positioned to correct from within.

6.3 The 2020 Community Pharmacists Study: Drug Information, Pharmaceutical Care and a Zero Competency Baseline

A second window into CPD needs in Qatar came from the mixed-methods study by Al-Sulaiti, Fares, Awaisu, and Kheir (2021), published in the International Quarterly of Community Health Education, which targeted community pharmacists specifically. Community pharmacists in Qatar operate in a demanding and frequently undervalued environment: they are, as the study noted, one hundred percent expatriates, trained in Middle Eastern and Asian educational systems that vary substantially in their clinical orientation, and working in a private sector where pharmaceutical care services have historically been limited to the traditional dispensing role. The study used a questionnaire and an event diary, a methodological tool that allowed pharmacists to record real-time encounters and encounters from memory, alongside inferential statistical analysis of training priorities.

Drug information skills and pharmaceutical care processes were the most frequently identified topics for CPD programme inclusion. More strikingly, not a single community pharmacist in the study considered themselves competent in any core area of pharmacy practice, a finding that the researchers described with understandable caution, given the concerns about self-report reliability that the earlier JCEHP paper had raised. Were these pharmacists accurately recognising genuine competency gaps, or were they performing a kind of professional modesty that the survey instrument invited? The answer is almost certainly that both dynamics were at play simultaneously, which is precisely what makes self-report data so difficult to interpret.

The event diary data, which captured pharmacists' own observations of their patient encounters in real time rather than their retrospective self-assessments of competence, added a dimension that questionnaire-only studies cannot reach. Pharmacists who recorded their encounters identified communication skills and medication safety as the areas in which they most frequently felt underprepared in practice, a finding that aligned with the observer assessments in the JCEHP study more closely than with the pharmacists' own questionnaire responses. There is something instructive in this: pharmacists who were asked what they needed in the abstract gave different answers from pharmacists who were asked to record what they actually struggled with in practice. The closer the needs assessment method came to the reality of practice, the more honestly it captured the gap.

The study identified a CPD programme architecture in response to these findings, one that prioritised patient-centred competencies and communication skills over the product-focused and fact-intensive topics that pharmacists themselves had initially foregrounded. Whether such a programme was subsequently designed and delivered, and whether it changed anything in the practice environment, is a question that the published literature has not yet answered for this specific cohort.

6.4 A Contradiction That Rewards Examination: Overestimation, Underestimation and What the Discrepancy Actually Reveals?

A careful reader of the two needs assessment studies described in this chapter will notice something that deserves direct confrontation rather than a quiet footnote: they appear to point in opposite directions.

The JCEHP triangulation study (Kheir, Al-Ismail and Al-Nakeeb, 2017) found that pharmacists overestimated their competence relative to external observers, the classic

Dunning–Kruger direction. Sixty-five percent of pharmacists described themselves as fully or reasonably satisfied with their competency level; only 21% of observing students and 14% of managers agreed. The bias ran consistently upward: pharmacists rated themselves higher than the evidence warranted.

The Al-Sulaiti et al. (2021) study of community pharmacists found precisely the opposite: not a single pharmacist in the study considered themselves competent in any core area of pharmacy practice. The direction of bias, if any existed, ran consistently downward.

Two studies, the same country, the same profession, the same methodology of self-report and opposite findings. How should this be reconciled?

The easy answer is to invoke methodological caution about self-report in both directions and move on. That would be the wrong response, both analytically and intellectually. The apparent contradiction is, in fact, one of the most interesting and informative things our research group's CPD work produced, because when examined carefully it points toward something important about the relationship between professional identity, practice environment and self-perception.

6.5 The Strongest Explanation: These Were not Comparable Populations

The JCEHP study sampled primarily from hospital and primary healthcare pharmacists, with the majority working in the public hospital sector. The Al-Sulaiti study targeted community pharmacists exclusively. In Qatar, and across the Gulf region more broadly, these two groups inhabit fundamentally different professional worlds, and the difference runs deeper than setting.

Hospital pharmacists in Qatar, particularly those working in Hamad Medical Corporation's Joint Commission International-accredited hospitals, operate within clinical environments that expect, support and reward pharmaceutical care practice. They work alongside physicians and nurses in clinical teams, conduct medication reconciliation, identify drug-related problems and participate in patient-centred activities. Their professional identity is shaped daily by an environment that treats them as clinicians. Even pharmacists who do not fully meet the standards of pharmaceutical care practice work in settings where that standard is visible, aspired to, and occasionally achieved. For this group, overestimation of competence is the predictable consequence of a clinical professional identity operating in an affirming environment.

Community pharmacists in Qatar faced a fundamentally different reality. As described in Chaps. 1 and 5 of this book, community pharmacy in Qatar, as in most of the MENA region and across low- and middle-income countries more broadly, remains structurally constrained to a product-focused dispensing role. The pharmacy law concerned itself with registration, premises and controlled drugs rather than professional mandate. Remuneration rewarded product sales rather than counselling or care planning. The public regarded community pharmacists primarily as medicine vendors. Commercial throughput was the dominant operational priority. Kheir (2025) framed this as the paradox of community pharmacy in low- and middle-income countries: pharmacies that are the most accessible points of contact in the healthcare system, staffed by professionals who are increasingly well-educated, yet structurally constrained to roles that prevent them from using what they know.

In this environment, a community pharmacist who has been trained to aspire to pharmaceutical care practice, and many of those sampled in the Al-Sulaiti study had attended Qatar University's CPD programmes, arrives at work each day in a state of chronic professional dissonance. They know what pharmaceutical care should look like. They see the gap between that ideal and their daily reality. And that gap is expressed, in a self-assessment instrument, as perceived incompetence.

This is not humility. It is a structurally produced self-perception, and recent research from our group sheds light on its psychological underpinnings. The Abd Al Magied et al. (2025) study of professional self-actualisation among UAE pharmacists across practice settings found that self-actualisation scores were significantly higher in hospital than in community settings, and that professional fulfilment correlated strongly with a supportive work environment ($r = 0.744$). The working environment does not merely shape what pharmacists can do. It shapes how they see themselves and how high they aim. A community pharmacist whose practice environment sends the daily message that their professional role is to count tablets and process transactions will, over time, internalise a professional self-concept calibrated to that environment rather than to the ideals of pharmaceutical care. When asked whether they consider themselves competent in pharmaceutical care practice, the honest answer, shaped by daily experience of that gap, was no.

6.6 The Secondary Explanations That Add Texture

Three secondary factors complement the population difference without displacing it as the primary explanation.

Different instruments may have set different standards. The JCEHP study used NAPRA competency domains, a Canadian regulatory framework defined in terms of professional role and function. The Al-Sulaiti instrument was calibrated to pharmaceutical care practice standards that are, in some respects, more demanding. A pharmacist who rates themselves as reasonably competent in "providing drug information" under a NAPRA framework may simultaneously rate themselves as incompetent in "pharmaceutical care delivery" under a more demanding instrument. These constructs are not equivalent, and they need not produce the same self-assessment.

Social desirability pressures may have operated differently across the two contexts. In the JCEHP study, pharmacists assessed by an academic institution may have felt professional competence was expected of them. Community pharmacists in the Al-Sulaiti study, attending an exercise explicitly designed to identify CPD needs, faced the opposite social pressure: rating oneself as competent would implicitly deny the need for the CPD being offered.

Finally, there is a dimension of the Dunning–Kruger framework operating in an unexpected direction. The competence–confidence curve predicts that people with very limited knowledge overestimate their abilities. But it also describes a zone of genuine expertise in which practitioners, having developed a sophisticated understanding of what competence truly requires, become more accurate, and sometimes more conservative, in their self-assessments. Community pharmacists who had attended pharmaceutical care CPD programmes and therefore understood what the standard actually demands may, paradoxically, have been demonstrating a more sophisticated self-awareness, not a less accurate one.

6.7 What the Contradiction Teaches?

Taken together, these explanations converge on a conclusion that the CPD research literature has not adequately articulated: self-assessed competence is not a stable psychological construct that measures approximately the same thing across contexts. It is a contextually produced perception that reflects practice environment, professional identity, instrument design and the degree to which a practitioner has been exposed to a demanding standard of practice against which to measure themselves.

The apparent contradiction between the two studies is therefore not a methodological embarrassment. It is a finding. It tells us that hospital pharmacists in the Gulf, working in affirming clinical environments, tend to overestimate their competence. It tells us that community pharmacists, working in environments that structurally contradict their professional training, tend to accurately perceive a gap between their potential and their practice that the environment prevents them from closing. Both are problems. Both have different implications for CPD design. And neither would have been visible without the apparent contradiction that researchers might otherwise have tried to explain away rather than take seriously.

6.8 The Critical Turn: Does CPD Actually Change What Pharmacists Do?

Both of the studies described above addressed the front end of the CPD problem: what do pharmacists need, and how reliably can they tell us? Neither addressed the back end, which is, in some respects, the more important question: once training is delivered, does it change what pharmacists do with patients? The study by Wilbur et al. (2017), published in the International Journal of Clinical Pharmacy, addressed this question directly, and the answer it produced was considerably more nuanced than the CPD literature typically celebrates.

The study developed and delivered a structured CPD programme for community pharmacists in Qatar on the management of diabetes patients who intended to fast during Ramadan. This is not a marginal clinical scenario in the Qatari context. Ramadan fasting is both an important religious obligation and a significant health risk for the roughly 43% of patients with type 2 diabetes who fast despite medical advice to the contrary. Pharmacists are ideally positioned to provide medication adjustment guidance, risk stratification and patient education at this critical juncture: they are accessible, trusted for over-the-counter guidance, and in regular contact with patients purchasing diabetes medications. The CPD programme was carefully designed, using standardised patient training and a combination of didactic, case-based and interactive learning strategies that reflect best practice in health professions education. Forty-one pharmacists attended.

The question the research addressed was not whether the programme improved pharmacists' knowledge, it almost certainly did, as virtually every well-designed educational intervention improves knowledge scores in the short term. The question was whether pharmacists who attended actually incorporated the new knowledge and skills into their patient interactions in the 3 weeks leading up to and during Ramadan. To answer this, the research team used an innovative pharmacist diary methodology: participating pharmacists recorded their encounters in real time using a mobile application, generating a naturalistic dataset of what actually happened when trained pharmacists tried to apply new knowledge in their practice environments.

Thirty-five of the forty-one attending pharmacists made at least one diary entry. What they recorded was illuminating and, if read carefully, sobering. Three factors shaped pharmacists' ability to use what they had learned: situational factors, patient factors, and pharmacist factors. Situational factors included the pharmacy's location, parking availability affecting how rushed customers felt, and the time of day. Patient factors included language barriers, patient age and receptivity, and the frequent reality that it was a family member or driver rather than the patient themselves who came to collect medications. Pharmacist factors included confidence with specific aspects of the guidance and the presence or absence of pre-existing relationships with patients.

Of these three, patient-related factors dominated. Patient reception was the most consistently reported influence on whether pharmacists attempted counselling and whether those attempts succeeded. Positive patient interactions encouraged pharmacists to continue engaging; difficult encounters, patients who were dismissive, who preferred to take advice only from physicians, or who suspected the pharmacist of commercial motives, functioned as powerful negative reinforcing stimuli that reduced willingness to initiate subsequent conversations. The social cognitive theory framework the researchers applied to these findings is instructive: behaviour is not determined by knowledge alone but by the dynamic interaction between knowledge, personal factors and the social environment. A pharmacist who knows how to counsel a fasting diabetes patient but who has learned, through repeated negative encounters, that such counselling is unwelcome in their specific practice context, will rationally invest their limited relational capital elsewhere.

The study's conclusion was measured but clear: in a Middle Eastern practice setting, environmental factors play a considerable role in pharmacists' ability to engage in public health care, and continuing education for health professionals must be closely aligned with the realities of practice and purposefully designed to account for those realities. This is not a new finding in the health professions education literature, the futility of passive CPD for changing behaviour has been documented since the 1990s, but it is a finding that had not previously been demonstrated in the Qatar pharmacy context with this level of methodological sophistication and ecological validity. The pharmacists who attended this programme were not failing because the training was poor. They were encountering the structural limits of what CPD alone can achieve when the practice environment it is designed to change has not itself been reformed.

This finding reframes the CPD problem in a way that the needs assessment literature rarely acknowledges. The question is not just what pharmacists need to know, or how reliably they can identify those needs, or how effectively training can address them. The deeper question is what the practice environment will allow pharmacists to do with what they know. A CPD programme that increases pharmacist knowledge by thirty percent and changes pharmacist behaviour by three percent is not a failure of education. It is a signal about the environment.

6.9 Looking Forward: Microcredentials and the Future Architecture of CPD

The limitations of traditional CPD delivery, conference attendance, workshop participation, passive didactic events, have been documented repeatedly in the health professions education literature. The challenge is not that pharmacists resist learning but that the formats through which learning has historically been delivered are poorly suited to the realities of a busy clinical workforce: inflexible timing, high cost, geographic concentration in urban centres, poor alignment with individual learning needs and limited capacity for personalisation. The question of what alternative architectures might better serve the profession's learning needs led our research group, in 2022, to a qualitative exploration of microcredentials as a potential CPD innovation.

The Lok et al. (2022) study, published in BMC Medical Education, conducted semi-structured telephone interviews with eleven pharmacy practitioners, policymakers and academics across seven countries, such as Egypt, Brazil, Kuwait, China, New Zealand, the United Kingdom and Japan, to explore perceptions of microcredentials as a CPD mechanism. Microcredentials are short, self-paced courses that certify the achievement of specific skills or knowledge, typically verified through a digital badge. They have attracted substantial interest across education sectors as a way of disaggregating learning into smaller, more accessible units that can be pursued flexibly, documented verifiably and accumulated progressively.

Participants across contexts identified several genuine advantages. Microcredentials offered flexibility in timing and location that traditional CPD formats could not match. They could be tailored to individual knowledge gaps rather than requiring attendance at generalist programmes designed for average needs. They could be delivered at lower cost than postgraduate certificates while providing verifiable evidence of competency acquisition. Several participants noted that the digital badging infrastructure associated with microcredentials offered a transparency about specific competencies that conventional degree designations could not provide: an employer looking at a pharmacist's profile of digital badges could see not just that the pharmacist had a degree or a CPD certificate, but specifically which competencies they had demonstrated and how they had been assessed.

Concerns were also consistently identified. Recognition was the most frequently cited challenge: microcredentials are a new concept, and many employers, professional bodies and regulatory authorities have not yet established frameworks for evaluating or crediting them. The risk that microcredentials might substitute for more substantial postgraduate learning, rather than complementing it, was raised by several participants. The quality and rigour of assessment within microcredentials was a genuine concern, whether a short course, however, well designed, could assess competency with the reliability that clinical practice requires. And the motivational challenge was real: pharmacists who are not required by their regulatory framework to engage in continuing education have limited external incentive to pursue microcredentials, regardless of how flexibly they are delivered.

The study was exploratory and explicitly so: it did not aim to test whether microcredentials work as CPD tools, because no pharmacy microcredentials existed in sufficient number at the time of the research to evaluate. It aimed to understand what the profession's own stakeholders thought about the concept, and what conditions would need to be in place for microcredentials to fulfil their potential. Those conditions, as the research identified them, included robust institutional partnerships between universities and practice settings to ensure curricular relevance, legislative and regulatory frameworks that recognised microcredentials as legitimate CPD contributions, quality assurance mechanisms that could withstand professional scrutiny, and institutional commitment from pharmacy schools to develop and sustain programme offerings that were genuinely calibrated to practice needs rather than commercially driven.

The connection to the earlier studies in this chapter is direct. If traditional CPD delivery is ineffective at changing practice because it is insufficiently aligned with practice realities, and if the barriers to CPD engagement include cost, inflexibility and poor match between standardised programme content and individual learning needs, then microcredentials represent at least a plausible architectural response to some of those problems. Whether they can address the deeper environmental barrier identified by the Wilbur et al. study, the practice environment that determines whether any training translates into behaviour change, is a different and more fundamental question that microcredentials alone cannot answer.

6.10 A Set of Critical Reflections

Looking back at this body of work, several things become clear that did not feel quite as clear at the time each study was conducted.

The first is that the needs assessment methodology we used, including the triangulation approach that was its most sophisticated expression, was addressing the wrong end of the CPD problem with the wrong tools. The JCEHP paper demonstrated that self-report is unreliable, which is a useful finding, but the triangulation solution it proposed, comparing self-report with student and manager observations, did not resolve the core difficulty. What it revealed was a disagreement between different perspectives, each of which carried its own biases, and offered no reliable way to adjudicate between them. The more important lesson from that study, which I did not fully articulate at the time, is that competency needs assessments in pharmacy practice are only meaningful if they are anchored to clear, shared, externally validated standards of what competent pharmaceutical care practice actually looks like. Without that anchor, we are measuring opinions about competence rather than competence itself.

The second reflection is about the Wilbur et al. study. I was a co-author on that paper, and the finding about environmental barriers to CPD translation was not a surprise, the literature had been saying something similar for years. What was clarifying about working with data from a naturalistic pharmacist diary in a specific practice context was seeing how immediate and granular those barriers are. It is not that pharmacists lack motivation or that training fails to produce knowledge. It is that a patient who says "just give me my medicine" in response to a counselling attempt creates a reinforcement signal that shapes subsequent behaviour more powerfully than a morning's CPD training can counteract. The practice environment trains pharmacists too, continuously, powerfully and in directions that are frequently opposite to what CPD is trying to achieve.

The third reflection concerns what our research group's work on CPD did not address, and should have. None of the studies in this chapter, including those I led, measured patient outcomes. We measured knowledge, self-perceived competence, observer-perceived competence and self-reported behaviour. We did not measure whether patients of pharmacists who had attended our CPD programmes experienced fewer medication-related problems, had better-controlled diabetes, or reported better quality of life. This is the measurement gap that the entire CPD research field has struggled with, not just in pharmacy and not just in Qatar, but the absence of that evidence from our own work is an honest limitation I want to name. Without patient outcome data, we cannot say with confidence that our CPD programmes did what they were designed to do. We can say that pharmacists gained knowledge, that some of them tried to apply it, and that many of them encountered barriers when they did. Whether any of that ultimately helped, or impacted, patients is a question we did not answer.

The fourth reflection is about the professional environment that all of this CPD activity was trying to work within. Continuing professional development, however, well designed, cannot substitute for the structural conditions that enable pharmaceutical care: regulatory frameworks that mandate and remunerate it, clinical governance systems that hold pharmacists accountable for it, practice environments that give them the time, space and patient relationships to provide it. Qatar's pharmacy landscape, during the period this research was conducted, had some of those conditions in the hospital sector and very few of them in the community sector. CPD investments in community pharmacist competence were, in that context, investments in building capacity that the practice environment could not fully absorb. Knowing that more clearly at the outset would not have made the CPD work less important, but it would have made it more honest about what it could and could not achieve.

6.11 Research Agenda Note

The body of work described in this chapter leaves five questions that the next generation of researchers in pharmacy CPD and professional development will need to address if the field is to make genuine progress.

First: what does a valid, reliable, and externally anchored assessment of pharmacist CPD needs actually look like? The triangulation approach demonstrated the limitations of self-report without providing a workable alternative. Developing needs assessment methodologies that are grounded in externally validated competency standards, embedded in routine professional practice rather than administered as surveys, and capable of distinguishing between wants and genuine needs, without becoming so burdensome that practitioners will not engage with them, is arguably the foundational methodological challenge in this field.

Second: under what conditions does CPD actually change patient-relevant outcomes? The gap between knowledge acquisition and behaviour change, and between behaviour change and patient outcomes, has been documented at the level of systematic reviews and meta-analyses but remains poorly characterised at the level of specific CPD interventions in specific practice environments. We need studies that follow the causal chain from CPD programme design through to pharmacist behaviour through to patient experience, with appropriate attention to the mediating role of the practice environment, rather than stopping at post-programme knowledge assessment.

Third: what practice environment conditions are necessary and sufficient for CPD to translate into sustained behaviour change? Wilbur et al. (2017) identified patient reception as a dominant environmental factor, but that was a single study in a single setting during a single Ramadan cycle. Understanding the relative weight of different environmental mediators, regulatory framework, remuneration structure, clinical governance, patient trust, interdisciplinary relationships, workplace culture and how they interact with CPD investment requires sustained longitudinal research that the field has not yet produced.

Fourth: can microcredentials deliver on their potential as a CPD architecture for pharmacy, and if so, what governance and quality assurance structures are required? The Lok et al. (2022) study identified the conditions, but conditions are not outcomes. The next step is to design, deliver and rigorously evaluate microcredential programmes in pharmacy CPD programs, with outcome measures that go beyond participant satisfaction and short-term knowledge scores to include competency demonstration, behaviour change in practice, and ultimately patient outcomes.

Fifth: how should CPD in pharmacy be redesigned for heterogeneous, expatriate-dominated workforces in rapidly developing healthcare systems? The Qatar context, with its 100% expatriate community pharmacy workforce trained across multiple educational systems with vastly different clinical orientations, is not unique: similar dynamics operate in the UAE, Kuwait, Saudi Arabia and across much of the Gulf healthcare workforce. Standard CPD frameworks designed for domestically trained, culturally homogeneous workforces operating in stable regulatory environments may not be adequate tools for this context. Designing CPD that is calibrated to workforce heterogeneity, that starts from where practitioners actually are, not where a standardised competency framework assumes they should be, is a research and design challenge that the MENA pharmacy CPD literature has barely begun to address.[1]

References

Abd Al Magied A, Beyene K, Arafa E, Elnour A, Kheir N (2025) Professional self-actualisation of pharmacists in the United Arab Emirates: a pilot study. J Pharm Policy Pract 18(1):2443524*

Al-Sulaiti F, Fares H, Awaisu A, Kheir N (2021) Continuing professional development needs of community pharmacists in Qatar: a mixed-methods approach. Int Q Community Health Educ 41(3):285–292*

Kheir N (2025) The paradox of community pharmacy practice in low- and middle-income countries (LMICs). J Pharm Policy Pract 18(1):2475082*

Kheir N, Al-Ismail MS, Al-Nakeeb R (2017) Can source triangulation be used to overcome limitations of self-assessments? Assessing educational needs and professional competence of pharmacists practicing in Qatar. J Contin Educ Health Professions 37(2):83–89*

Lok P, Beyene K, Awaisu A, Woods D, Kheir N (2022) Microcredentials training in pharmacy practice and education: an exploratory study of its viability and pharmacists' professional needs. BMC Med Educ 22:332*

Wilbur K, Shabana S, Maraghi F, ElMubark A, Kheir N (2017) An evaluation of the translation of continuing education into diabetes public health care by pharmacists. Int J Clin Pharm 39(4):774–782*

[1] Publications by the author of this book are marked with an asterisk (*) in references.

Chapter 7
Building Research Capacity: Can You Teach a Pharmacist to Think Like a Scientist?

7.1 The Anchor Publication

This chapter is built around a study our team designed and conducted at Hamad Medical Corporation in Qatar, evaluating a structured research capacity-building programme for hospital pharmacists and subsequently published in the Journal of Pharmaceutical Health Services Research (Awaisu et al. 2015). It is a paper about postgraduate professional development, about what happens when practising pharmacists are brought back into a learning environment and asked to acquire research skills they did not develop during their undergraduate formation. But this chapter also tells a parallel story, one that the published paper does not tell, about what it looks like to build research capacity at the undergraduate level, to embed research participation in the pharmacy curriculum itself, so that graduates arrive in their professional careers already possessing the foundational habits of scientific inquiry. These two stories, the postgraduate HMC programme and the undergraduate UREP model at Qatar University, represent different responses to the same problem, and reading them together reveals more about research capacity building in the Gulf than either story alone.

7.2 The Foundational Tension

There is a foundational tension at the heart of pharmacy practice research in the developing world that presents itself differently depending on where you sit. From the perspective of a health system planner, the tension is between the urgent clinical need for local evidence and the absence of local researchers capable of generating it. From the perspective of a pharmacy educator, the tension is between an undergraduate curriculum already crowded with pharmacological, clinical and professional content and the additional burden of research training that effective evidence-based practice

N. Kheir, *Medicines, Patients, and the Gaps Between*,
https://doi.org/10.1007/978-981-92-5395-1_7

requires. From the perspective of a practising pharmacist, the tension is between the daily demands of clinical work, which in most Gulf settings leave no protected time for research activity, and the intellectual aspiration to contribute to the knowledge base of the profession.

These three tensions are related but distinct, and they require different responses. The HMC programme our team developed was designed primarily to address the first and third tensions: practising hospital pharmacists with clinical responsibilities and no protected research time were brought into a structured learning programme that developed their research knowledge and self-perceived competence through a combination of didactic instruction and hands-on project work (Awaisu et al. 2015). The Undergraduate Research Experience Program (UREP) a national research funding initiative in Qatar was designed to address the second tension: by embedding funded research participation in the undergraduate curriculum, it created a pathway through which pharmacy students could acquire genuine research experience without requiring additional curriculum time, because the research activity was the curriculum.

7.3 The HMC Programme: What It Did and What It Found?

A structured research capacity-building programme our team designed and delivered to pharmacists at Hamad Medical Corporation, Qatar's primary public health system provider, across two specialised tertiary care hospitals, was subsequently evaluated and published in the Journal of Pharmaceutical Health Services Research (Awaisu et al. 2015). The programme combined didactic instruction in research methodology with supervised hands-on project work, covering research design, literature review, data collection and analysis and the preparation of research outputs for presentation and publication. Pre- and post-programme assessment measured changes in both objective research knowledge, using a validated knowledge test, and self-perceived research competence, using a structured self-assessment scale.

The findings were encouraging in their magnitude: participants showed statistically significant improvements in research knowledge and reported substantially increased confidence across multiple research competency domains, a result that validated the programme's core design (Awaisu et al. 2015). These are meaningful outcomes. Research capacity is not built by sending individual pharmacists to overseas universities and hoping they return with both the skills and the motivation to apply them locally. It is built by creating structured, contextually situated learning opportunities that develop competency within the practice environment where that competency will be used, and by embedding those opportunities in institutional cultures that value and reward research activity. The HMC programme did the first part of this well. Whether it succeeded in the second part, creating a lasting institutional culture of research inquiry within hospital pharmacy at HMC, is the harder and less answerable question.

A subsequent paper from the same institutional context, examining the perceptions of pharmacy students and alumni toward research after completing undergraduate research courses at Qatar University, found that alumni working in hospital settings perceived themselves to have significantly lower confidence in conducting research than those working in non-hospital settings, including academia and research institutes (Mukhalalati et al. 2022). This finding is consistent with the observation that conducting research is neither part of the job description of a hospital pharmacist nor a requirement for preregistration in Qatar or many other countries, meaning that engagement in research is not considered a priority in the hospital work environment regardless of training received. The structural conditions of the hospital pharmacy workplace, not the competence of individual pharmacists, remain the binding constraint on research productivity.

7.4 The UREP Model: Building Research into the Undergraduate Years

The Undergraduate Research Experience Program (UREP), administered currently by the Qatar Research, Development and Innovation Council, was established in 2006 by the Qatar National Research Fund (QNRF) as a nationally funded initiative to encourage undergraduate students and faculty members across Qatar's universities to strengthen the country's research infrastructure through participation in research projects. By its 17th cycle in November 2025, UREP had recognised over 5811 undergraduate students from eight universities across Qatar for their contributions to 1540 projects, of which 1289 had been completed across the programme's 19-year history (QRDI Council 2025). The programme explicitly serves both students and faculty, offering both groups the opportunity to build their research experience and academic portfolios, and it operates in deliberate alignment with Qatar National Vision 2030, which aspires to position Qatar as a global hub for talent in cutting-edge innovation, research, and development (QRDI Council 2025). This national strategic framing is significant: UREP was never simply a university enrichment activity. It was a nationally funded instrument of research capacity building, designed to populate Qatar's research ecosystem with trained investigators across all disciplines, including health sciences.

The College of Pharmacy at Qatar University adopted this programme as a deliberate and systematic feature of its undergraduate research strategy. Each year, our team applied to UREP with research proposals designed not only to address genuine clinical or pharmaceutical care questions but to provide genuine research experiences for the undergraduate students who participated in them. This was not research designed around student convenience. It was research designed to answer real questions, with students as genuine contributors and junior researchers to the investigative process rather than as assistants performing peripheral tasks. The result was that virtually all pharmacy students at QU-CPH participated in at least one UREP-funded research project during their undergraduate studies, and more than 80% of graduates had their names on peer-reviewed publications by the time they completed their degree.

This outcome is remarkable by any international benchmark. Most pharmacy programmes, including highly regarded programmes in North America and Europe, do not routinely produce graduates with peer-reviewed publications. The PharmD programmes that most explicitly incorporate research training typically do so through elective research tracks or senior capstone projects that produce institutional reports or conference presentations rather than submitted manuscripts. At QU-CPH, peer-reviewed publication was not the exceptional achievement of a research-track minority but the normal outcome of a standard undergraduate education, because the UREP programme provided the funding, the mentorship and the motivational structure that converted undergraduate research participation into publishable evidence.

The scholarly literature examining this model confirms both its value and its complexity. A Frontiers in Medicine study of QU pharmacy students and alumni found that over 91% of respondents had participated in a UREP project during their undergraduate degree, and that participation was associated with significantly higher research confidence and positive attitudes toward the value of research for pharmacy practice (Mukhalalati et al. 2022). Faculty members who taught in the programme observed that students who had completed UREP projects entered subsequent research courses with demonstrably stronger baseline knowledge and confidence than those who had not, precisely because the earlier research experience had already given them a working vocabulary, a methodological orientation and a sense of what research actually demands of its practitioners (Mukhalalati et al. 2022).

7.5 Two Models, One Problem: Complementary Responses to the Capacity Gap

The HMC programme and the UREP model represent different but complementary strategies for closing the same gap: the shortage of pharmacy practitioners in Qatar who possess both the will and the competence to generate the local evidence base that the profession needs. The HMC programme addresses the gap retrospectively, by developing research skills in pharmacists who are already practising and who have entered their careers without adequate research formation. The UREP model addresses the gap prospectively, by building research competence into the undergraduate formation of pharmacists before they enter practice, so that the research-capable pharmacist becomes the norm rather than the exception.

Neither strategy alone is sufficient. The UREP graduates who enter hospital pharmacy and find no protected time, no research infrastructure and no institutional expectation of research activity will not sustain their research capabilities regardless of how well their undergraduate formation prepared them. The HMC programme participants who return to a pharmacy department that does not value research productivity, that does not create opportunities for funded projects or submission of manuscripts, and that assesses performance entirely on clinical throughput will not convert their newly acquired knowledge into research outputs. Capacity building is not an individual intervention. It is a systemic change that requires alignment between education, institutional culture, professional expectation and dedicated resources at every level.

7.6 What the Field Did with These Publications

Our HMC capacity-building paper (Awaisu et al. 2015) has been cited in subsequent regional research capacity-building literature and in papers examining the evidence base for pharmacy practice research training programmes in the Middle East and North Africa. It was cited in the Mukhalalati et al. (2022) Frontiers in Medicine study of undergraduate research at QU as a complementary model of postgraduate research capacity development, with the authors explicitly noting the parallel between our programme's findings on hospital pharmacist research confidence and their own findings on the relatively lower research confidence of alumni working in hospital settings. This cross-citation between the undergraduate and postgraduate models represents a productive scholarly conversation about the different mechanisms and different stages at which research capacity needs to be built, and about the institutional conditions that either enable or constrain its development.

The UREP model itself has not, to my knowledge, been examined in a single comprehensive publication that documents its pharmacy-specific outcomes across the full history of QU's programme participation, though related work on student and faculty perceptions of undergraduate research courses at QU has been published (Mukhalalati et al., 2022). That documentation gap is itself significant: the most important evidence of the model's impact, the proportion of graduates with peer-reviewed publications, the research topics that undergraduate projects addressed, the clinical and policy questions they contributed to answering, and the subsequent career trajectories of graduates who participated, exists in institutional records and in the publication histories of individual graduates but has not been assembled into a published account that the regional or international literature can cite. Writing that account is an unfinished obligation, and one that those of us who were part of that story are uniquely positioned to fulfil.

7.7 The Gap the Research Left Open

The most significant limitation of our HMC programme evaluation (Awaisu et al. 2015) is the one that most programme evaluations share: it measured outcomes at the immediate post-programme stage rather than at the point that matters most, which is whether participants went on to conduct, complete and publish research in the years following the programme. Changes in knowledge test scores and self-confidence ratings at programme completion are necessary evidence that the training worked as education. They are insufficient evidence that the training worked as capacity building, because capacity building is only demonstrated when the capacity is actually used. The longitudinal follow-up study that would answer the question of sustained impact has not been published.

A second gap is the absence, in both the HMC programme and the UREP model, of systematic attention to the institutional conditions that either sustain or erode research capacity after initial development. Building research skills in an individual pharmacist is a necessary but insufficient condition for building a research-active pharmacy profession. The necessary sufficient condition is an institutional environment that creates space for research activity, recognises and rewards it in performance assessment frameworks, provides access to funding and mentorship and connects individual researchers to a community of scholarly peers. That environment does not currently exist uniformly in the region's hospital pharmacy sector or in its community pharmacy sector, and its absence is the most important factor limiting the translation of the region's growing research training investment into published evidence that improves patient care.

7.8 Research Agenda Note

The capacity-building programmes documented in this chapter point toward five open questions that represent the most important unfinished work on research capacity in the region's pharmacy profession.

First: do pharmacists who complete research training go on to conduct, complete and publish research in the years that follow? The HMC programme evaluation measured knowledge and confidence at programme completion; the longitudinal follow-up that would demonstrate capacity in use has not been published. A cohort study tracing the research output of HMC programme participants and UREP alumni over 5–10 years is the study this chapter's own honesty demands.

Second: which institutional conditions sustain research productivity after training, and which erode it? Building skills in individuals is necessary but insufficient. Implementation studies testing specific organisational interventions, protected research time, funded infrastructure, mentorship access and performance frameworks that recognise research activity, would identify the environmental changes that convert trained individuals into a research-active profession.

Third: does undergraduate research experience predict career-long research engagement? The UREP model rests on the premise that early exposure shapes professional identity. Now in its 19th year, the programme has produced enough alumni for that premise to be tested empirically, through career-tracking studies comparing UREP participants with matched non-participants on subsequent research involvement, postgraduate study and publication.

Fourth: which capacity-building design works best for practising pharmacists? Intensive workshop programmes of the HMC type, longitudinal mentorship models and embedded practice-based research networks make different assumptions about how working professionals learn to do research. Comparative evaluations of these models, with sustained research activity rather than post-programme test scores as the endpoint, would give the region's institutions an evidence base for their training investments.

Fifth: how should locally generated research capacity be connected to locally defined research priorities? Capacity without an agenda risks producing more of the descriptive research this book critiques. Research examining how national frameworks of the kind the QRDI Council represents can align trained pharmacist researchers with the health system's actual evidence needs would close the loop between building capacity and using it where it matters.

7.9 What Remains?

The question posed in this chapter's title, Can You Teach a Pharmacist to Think like a Scientist? Has a straightforward answer: yes, demonstrably, at both the undergraduate and postgraduate levels, and the evidence from both the UREP model and our HMC programme supports that conclusion. The harder question, which neither programme has yet answered, is whether a pharmacist who has been taught to think like a scientist will continue to do so in a practice environment that was not designed with scientific inquiry in mind.

Answering that harder question requires the next generation of research capacity-building work in the Gulf to move beyond training programme evaluation and into implementation science: studies that examine what institutional conditions enable or constrain sustained research productivity among trained pharmacists, that test specific organisational interventions, including protected research time, funded research infrastructure and performance frameworks that recognise research activity, and that measure their impact on the volume and quality of locally generated evidence. Building those conditions is a longer and more complex project than designing a research training programme. But it is the project that the profession's evidence needs require, and it is the project that the capacity-building work described in this chapter, at HMC and at Qatar University, was always pointing toward.

The UREP programme itself, now in its nineteenth year and still growing, offers one model of what sustained national investment in undergraduate research capacity looks like over the long arc of institution building. Since its inception in 2006, it has supported 1540 projects and recognised 5811 students across Qatar's universities, a scale of investment that reflects a genuine national commitment to making research participation a normal feature of undergraduate education rather than an elite exception (QRDI Council 2025). The pharmacy profession in the Gulf would benefit from an equivalent commitment at the practice level: sustained, nationally funded investment in the conditions that allow trained researchers to do research, not just in the training itself.[1]

References

Awaisu A, Kheir N, Alrowashdeh HA, Allouch SN, Jebara T, Zaidan M, Mohamed Ibrahim MI (2015) Impact of a pharmacy practice research capacity-building programme on improving the research abilities of pharmacists at two specialised tertiary care hospitals in Qatar: a preliminary study. J Pharm Health Serv Res 6(3):155–164*

Mukhalalati B, Elshami S, Adlan O, Elshazly M, Awaisu A, Stewart D, Al-Badriyeh D, Alali F (2022) Perceptions and experiences of undergraduate pharmacy students and alumni toward research after exposure to undergraduate research courses. Front Med 9:988908

QRDI Council (2025) QRDI Council celebrates young scholars driving Qatar's research future at the 17th UREP and 9th BRIO Awards. https://qrdi.org.qa/en-US/News-Details/Id/186

[1] Publications by the author of this book are marked with an asterisk (*) in references.

Chapter 8
Adherence, Barriers and the Chronic Disease Compact

8.1 The Anchor Publications

This chapter is built around two publications from a sustained research programme on medication adherence in diabetes patients in Qatar, both arising from the doctoral work of a graduate student our team supervised. The first, Jaam et al. (2018a), published in Primary Care Diabetes, quantified the prevalence of non-adherence among patients with uncontrolled diabetes attending primary healthcare clinics and identified the patient-level and system-level barriers associated with poor adherence. The second, Jaam et al. (2018b), published in Patient Preference and Adherence, extended this work using a qualitative methodology to develop an in-depth understanding of those barriers by integrating the perspectives of both patients and healthcare providers. Together, these two publications represent a methodological progression from quantifying the problem to understanding it, and from the surface features of non-adherence to its lived meaning for the patients experiencing it. A third paper arising from the same programme, Jaam et al. (2017), published in Diabetes Research and Clinical Practice, was a systematic review of factors associated with medication adherence among patients with diabetes in the Middle East and North Africa region, providing the regional evidence base against which the Qatar-specific findings were interpreted.

8.2 The Ground the Research Stood On

Medication adherence in chronic disease is one of the most extensively studied problems in health services research, yet decades of investigation have produced surprisingly little change in the clinical picture. The foundational epidemiological picture has been stable for more than two decades: approximately half of patients with chronic conditions do not take their medications as prescribed, and the clinical and

N. Kheir, *Medicines, Patients, and the Gaps Between*,
https://doi.org/10.1007/978-981-92-5395-1_8

economic consequences, measured in disease progression, preventable hospitalisation and avoidable mortality, are substantial (Sabaté 2003). In the intervening years, the literature on adherence has expanded enormously without fundamentally shifting that picture. What has shifted, and only partially, is the conceptual framework within which non-adherence is understood.

The dominant framework for most of that history was essentially behavioural and motivational: patients did not adhere because they lacked knowledge, motivation or self-efficacy, and the remedy was therefore educational and psychological. That framework produced a generation of adherence interventions built around patient education, reminder systems, simplified regimens and motivational counselling, each of which demonstrated modest and variable effects in controlled conditions and smaller effects when evaluated in real clinical settings. The limitations of this approach became increasingly apparent as the literature accumulated: it placed the burden of change almost entirely on the patient, it treated non-adherence as a personal failing rather than a rational response to the demands of complex treatment regimens, and it consistently underestimated the role of system-level and structural factors in shaping what patients actually did with their medications. This is a typical example of deficit framing, known to obscure structural determinants of health and to influence policy in harmful ways (Link and Phelan 1995).

The shift toward a more patient-centred and structurally informed understanding of adherence was gradual and uneven, but by the time our team began designing the Qatar adherence studies in the early 2010s, the theoretical ground had shifted sufficiently to make a patient-centred, mixed-method approach both intellectually coherent and scientifically timely. The WHO report on adherence to long-term therapies had already argued that addressing adherence required a systems approach that attended to patient, provider, therapy, condition and health system factors simultaneously (Sabaté 2003). The concept of treatment burden, described in Chap. 2 of this book, had given researchers a framework for understanding why patients with high treatment demands made the clinical choices they did. What the Qatar context still lacked, at the time our studies were designed, was locally generated evidence on the specific barriers that Qatari and Qatar-based patients with uncontrolled diabetes were actually encountering, evidence that could not be assumed from international studies conducted in different healthcare systems, different cultural contexts and different patient populations.

Qatar's primary healthcare system at this time was undergoing significant development. Hamad Medical Corporation's primary healthcare clinics were the main institutional setting for the management of non-communicable diseases in the resident population, serving a patient base that was extraordinarily heterogeneous: Qatari nationals, who made up a minority of the population, alongside large communities of South Asian, Arab, Southeast Asian and African expatriate workers, each with different language backgrounds, different health beliefs, different relationships to formal healthcare and different social and economic circumstances. Designing adherence research in this environment required instruments and methods capable of capturing that heterogeneity, and it required an analytical framework that could distinguish between barriers operating at the level of the individual patient, the provider and the healthcare system, rather than collapsing them into a single undifferentiated adherence problem.

8.3 The Scale of the Problem

Diabetes is one of the most significant public health challenges facing Qatar and the broader Gulf region. Qatar has one of the highest age-standardised prevalences of type 2 diabetes in the world, and the complications of uncontrolled diabetes, including nephropathy, retinopathy, neuropathy and cardiovascular disease, impose an enormous burden on both patients and the health system. Despite this, the evidence base on medication adherence in Qatari diabetes patients was, at the time, these studies were conducted, thin. The studies our team conducted were among the first to quantify non-adherence specifically among the highest-risk group: patients with uncontrolled diabetes, defined by glycosylated haemoglobin A1c above 7% or fasting blood glucose above 130 mg/dL, who were already in regular contact with the healthcare system and receiving treatment.

The quantitative findings were stark. Among 260 patients with uncontrolled diabetes attending two primary healthcare clinics in Qatar, 73% were classified as non-adherent using the Adherence to Refill and Medications Scale in Diabetes (ARMS-D), a validated self-report measure (Jaam et al. 2018a). The ARMS-D, developed and validated in the United States and subsequently used across multiple cultural and linguistic contexts, captures two dimensions of adherence that are both clinically important and often measured separately in other instruments: adherence to refilling prescriptions and adherence to taking medications as directed. Its use in the Qatari context required confirmation of its linguistic and conceptual equivalence in Arabic, a methodological step that was undertaken as part of the study design and that built directly on the instrument validation experience described in Chap. 2 of this book. Non-adherent patients reported the majority of the predetermined barriers to medication adherence, with forgetfulness being the most commonly reported. Multivariate regression analysis identified age, ethnicity, education level, income level and baseline HbA1c as independent predictors of adherence, pointing directly to the social and demographic dimensions of adherence that purely clinical management frameworks were not addressing.

8.4 Beyond the Numbers: The Qualitative Study

The quantitative study established the scale and the correlates of non-adherence. What it could not do was explain, with the depth and specificity that clinical intervention requires, why patients were not adhering, what they understood about their medications, how they experienced the demands of their treatment regimen and what they believed their healthcare providers understood about those demands. The qualitative study (Jaam et al. 2018b) addressed this gap directly, using semi-structured face-to-face interviews with patients with uncontrolled diabetes and their healthcare providers, including physicians, pharmacists, nurses and dieticians, at the same two primary healthcare centres.

The findings revealed a landscape of barrier complexity that the quantitative study had measured but could not fully illuminate. Patient-level barriers included not only forgetfulness but also reliance on alternative medicine, fluctuating motivation and a sense of boredom with treatment that was partly a response to the monotony of chronic disease management and partly a reflection of inadequate engagement with the meaning and purpose of the medications being prescribed. Patients who had been told they needed to take metformin twice daily, and who did not understand why or who had been told about the long-term risks of uncontrolled diabetes but had never been helped to connect those risks to their own daily experience, were not failing to adhere out of ignorance. They were making rational, and deliberate, decisions in a context of insufficient clinical engagement with their individual circumstances. Health system barriers were equally prominent: brief consultation times that left patients with insufficient understanding of their treatment; inadequate patient education about the purpose of medications and the consequences of non-adherence and a fragmented care environment in which the pharmacist, the physician, the nurse and the dietician were each addressing different aspects of the patient's condition or its treatment, without an integrated framework for communicating the overall management plan.

A particularly important finding was the discrepancy between patients' and providers' understandings of why non-adherence was occurring. Healthcare providers tended to attribute non-adherence to patient knowledge deficits and motivational failures: patients did not understand the importance of their medications or they did not take their condition seriously enough. Patients, by contrast, described barriers that were more structural and experiential: the difficulty of fitting complex medication regimens into daily lives already crowded with work, family and competing obligations; the side effects that made taking medications uncomfortable; and the lack of adequate support from the health system for the practical challenges of long-term self-management. This mismatch between provider attribution and patient experience is not a trivial finding. It means that interventions designed around assumptions about why patients do not adhere will miss the actual barriers that need to be addressed, and will likely confirm the provider's pessimism about patient motivation rather than producing the improvement in adherence that a more accurately targeted intervention might achieve.

8.5 The Regional Systematic Review

Our team's systematic mixed studies review of factors associated with medication adherence among diabetes patients in the MENA region (Jaam et al. 2017) provided the contextual framework within which the Qatar-specific findings should be interpreted. The review, published in Diabetes Research and Clinical Practice, synthesised evidence from studies across the region and found that the determinants of non-adherence in the MENA context were broadly consistent with those identified internationally, but with important regional specificities that standard adherence frameworks did not adequately capture.

Three regional specificities deserve particular attention. The first was the role of religious beliefs and faith-based acceptance of illness. In several studies reviewed, patients described their diabetes as a test from God, an understanding that was not fatalistic in the passive sense but that shaped the emotional and motivational relationship to treatment in ways that secular clinical frameworks were poorly equipped to engage with. A clinician who interprets faith-based illness acceptance as resignation or non-compliance has misread both the patient and the cultural context, and the intervention they design in response to that misreading will be both clinically ineffective and culturally disrespectful. The second specificity was the influence of extended family structures on healthcare decision-making. In Gulf societies, healthcare decisions are frequently made within family systems rather than by individuals alone, and interventions that target only the patient, without attending to the family dynamics that shape whether medications are taken, which traditional remedies are used alongside or instead of prescribed medications, and whether the patient attends follow-up appointments, are addressing only part of the adherence picture. The third was the particular challenge of managing chronic disease in expatriate populations with limited continuity of care, where patients may change healthcare providers frequently, face language barriers in clinical consultations and lack the social infrastructure that sustained self-management requires.

8.6 From Research to the Classroom

The adherence research documented in this chapter did not remain confined to the peer-reviewed literature. It shaped, directly and deliberately, the way medication adherence was taught to pharmacy students at Qatar University's College of Pharmacy, and subsequently in the Master of Pharmacy Practice programme at the University of Waikato. The insight that drove this pedagogical connection was straightforward but important: a pharmacy student who understands adherence only as a patient behaviour problem will design interventions that are educationally adequate and clinically inadequate. A pharmacy student who understands adherence as the product of an interaction between a patient's circumstances, beliefs, and resources on one side, and the demands, structure and responsiveness of the healthcare system on the other, is equipped to ask the right questions before designing any intervention at all.

The provider-patient mismatch finding from Jaam et al. (2018b) became a teaching case in its own right. Students were presented with the finding, asked to reflect on why providers consistently attributed non-adherence to patient knowledge deficits when patients were consistently describing structural and experiential barriers, and then asked to design a brief clinical consultation that would elicit the patient's actual barriers rather than confirming the provider's assumptions. The exercise was not merely theoretical. It was grounded in data from the healthcare system in which many of those students would eventually practise, and it connected directly to the behaviour change frameworks described in Chap. 2 of this book. Understanding where a patient sits in the Transtheoretical Model of Change, and what specific beliefs and barriers are keeping them there, is exactly the clinical skill that the adherence research had shown was missing from provider-patient interactions in Qatar's primary care diabetes clinics. Teaching it required the evidence. The evidence came from the research.

8.7 What the Field Did with These Publications?

Jaam et al. (2018a) has been cited widely in subsequent regional diabetes adherence research and in systematic reviews of medication adherence in the Middle East. It was cited in a qualitative study of healthcare service delivery for uncontrolled diabetes in Qatar, published in 2025, which explicitly identified it as the foundational quantitative study of non-adherence in the Qatari primary care diabetes population and used its findings to frame the structural and service delivery gaps that the subsequent qualitative work explored. It was cited in a 2020 systematic review of adherence barriers in the Gulf, in a 2022 study of medication adherence predictors in Qatar, and in research from Indonesia, South Korea and Ethiopia that cited the Qatar primary care data as part of broader comparative analyses of diabetes adherence across different health system contexts. Jaam et al. (2017) has been cited as a foundational regional review in subsequent systematic reviews of diabetes adherence in the MENA region, in clinical practice guidelines for diabetes management in Gulf countries, and in educational programmes on medication adherence in pharmacy practice.

The breadth of this citation pattern is worth noting. A study of non-adherence in Qatar's primary healthcare clinics has been used to contextualise adherence research in Sub-Saharan Africa, East Asia and Southeast Asia. This is not because the specific barriers in those contexts mirror those in Qatar, but because the methodological approach, combining quantitative prevalence data with qualitative barrier analysis and a regional systematic review, provided a transferable template that subsequent researchers found useful. The research contributed to the field's methodological repertoire as well as to its substantive knowledge base.

8.8 The Gap the Research Left Open

The mixed-method design of the adherence programme represented a methodological advance over purely quantitative adherence surveys, but it still stopped short of the intervention evidence that the findings pointed toward. The mismatch between provider and patient understandings of non-adherence, identified so clearly in Jaam et al. (2018b), has direct implications for intervention design: if healthcare providers are educating patients based on incorrect assumptions about why they are not adhering, those educational interventions will be ineffective. Testing whether training providers to adopt a patient-centred perspective on adherence barriers, and restructuring the consultation to explicitly explore and address those barriers, improves adherence outcomes is a logical and clinically important next step that the research programme did not take.

A second gap is the absence of pharmacist involvement in the adherence picture that the studies described. The patients in these studies were attending primary healthcare clinics in Qatar, and they were interacting regularly with physicians, nurses and dieticians. The pharmacist, the healthcare professional with the most detailed knowledge of the medication regimen and its practical management demands, appears in the qualitative study only as one of several provider types, without a distinct or prominent role. In a healthcare system where medication-related burden, as documented in Chap. 2, is a significant driver of non-adherence, the pharmacist's potential role in identifying, discussing and helping to rationalise the burden of complex medication regimens was not examined. That is a gap with direct implications for pharmaceutical care practice and research in the Gulf primary care setting.

A third gap is longitudinal. Both the quantitative and qualitative studies captured the adherence experience at a single point in time. The barriers to adherence that patients described are not static: they change as disease progresses, as medication regimens are modified, as social and economic circumstances shift and as patients develop their own accumulated experience of managing a long-term condition. A patient who reports forgetfulness as their primary barrier at one consultation may be dealing with side effects, financial constraints or treatment fatigue at the next. Without longitudinal data, the research programme can describe the distribution of barriers in a cross-section of patients but cannot identify which patients are most likely to deteriorate, which barriers are most responsive to intervention or whether the provider-patient mismatch persists or narrows over time as clinical relationships develop.

8.9 Research Agenda Note

The adherence research programme documented in this chapter points toward five open questions that the existing evidence base has not yet answered and that represent the most important unfinished work in this field.

First: can a structured pharmacist-led medication review intervention, designed explicitly to identify and respond to patient-reported adherence barriers rather than provider-assumed ones, improve glycaemic control in patients with uncontrolled diabetes in primary healthcare settings? The qualitative evidence generated by studies such as those documented in this chapter is sufficient to justify a rigorously designed randomised controlled trial testing this question, with glycated haemoglobin as the primary outcome and patient-reported treatment burden and quality of life as secondary outcomes.

Second: how do adherence barriers differ across the major expatriate and cultural communities present in Gulf healthcare systems, and what culturally and linguistically adapted interventions are required to address population-specific barriers? The demographic heterogeneity of patient populations in these settings is one of the most clinically significant features of their primary healthcare context, and adherence interventions designed without attending to that heterogeneity will be effective for some patients and irrelevant for others.

Third: does integrating treatment burden assessment into routine diabetes consultations in primary care, using a validated treatment burden instrument such as the Living with Medicines Questionnaire, identify patients at elevated risk of non-adherence before clinical deterioration occurs? The connection between burden and adherence, established in Chap. 2 of this book, implies that burden assessment could function as a clinical early-warning tool but that implication has not been tested prospectively in the primary care setting.

Fourth: what is the longitudinal trajectory of medication adherence in patients with uncontrolled diabetes attending primary care systems, and which patient, provider and system factors predict sustained improvement versus continued non-adherence over a 2-year horizon? The cross-sectional design of Jaam et al. (2018a) established a prevalence estimate; a cohort study following similar patients over time could have established the dynamic picture that clinical management actually requires, and that opportunity remains open to future researchers in this field.

Fifth: can the provider-patient mismatch, like that documented in Jaam et al. (2018b), be addressed through a structured communication training programme for primary healthcare providers, and if so, does that training produce measurable improvements in the quality of adherence-related clinical consultations and in patient-reported experiences of care? These are training research questions as much as clinical research questions, and they sit at the intersection of pharmacy education, medical education and health services research in ways that make them particularly well suited to interdisciplinary investigation.

8.10 What Remains?

The adherence research agenda in Qatar and the wider MENA region has matured considerably, but it remains dominated by prevalence and barrier studies. What is needed now is the implementation evidence that the barrier studies have consistently implied: rigorously designed trials of specific, theory-informed interventions for reducing the barriers identified in studies such as Jaam et al. (2018a) and Jaam et al. (2018b), tested in the specific institutional context of Qatar's primary healthcare system, and measuring not just adherence rates but quality of life, treatment burden and patient experience outcomes. The conceptual framework developed in the Jaam et al. (2017) systematic review, and the patient-centred insight generated by the qualitative study, provide the theoretical foundation for those interventions. Building the evidence that they work is the most important unfinished task of this research programme, and it is a task that the research community in Qatar, with its established infrastructure, its validated instruments and its documented understanding of the patient population, is uniquely positioned to pursue.[1]

[1]Publications by the author of this book are marked with an asterisk (*) in references.

References

Jaam M, Ibrahim MIM, Kheir N, Awaisu A (2017) Factors associated with medication adherence among patients with diabetes in the Middle East and North Africa region: a systematic mixed studies review. Diabetes Res Clin Pract 129:1–15*

Jaam M, Mohamed Ibrahim MI, Kheir N, Hadi MA, Diab MI, Awaisu A (2018a) Assessing prevalence of and barriers to medication adherence in patients with uncontrolled diabetes attending primary healthcare clinics in Qatar. Prim Care Diabetes 12(2):116–125. *

Jaam M, Hadi MA, Kheir N, Mohamed Ibrahim MI, Diab MI, Al-Abdulla S, Awaisu A (2018b) A qualitative exploration of barriers to medication adherence among patients with uncontrolled diabetes in Qatar: integrating perspectives of patients and health care providers. Patient Prefer Adherence 12:2205–2216*

Link BG, Phelan J (1995) Social conditions as fundamental causes of disease. J Health Soc Behav 35(Extra Issue):80–94

Sabaté E (2003) Adherence to long-term therapies: evidence for action. World Health Organization, Geneva

Chapter 9
Listening to Caregivers: Autism, Burden and the Family Behind the Patient

9.1 The Anchor Publications

This chapter is built around two publications arising from a research programme our team developed at Qatar University, both funded by the Qatar National Research Fund through the UREP mechanism, and both addressing the same overlooked population: the caregivers of children with autism spectrum disorder in Qatar. The first, Kheir et al. (2012a), published in Autism, assessed the quality of life of caregivers of children with autism and compared it with that of caregivers of typically developing children. The second, Kheir et al. (2012b), published in BMC Research Notes, examined the specific concerns and considerations that shaped the caregiving experience in the Qatari cultural context, including caregivers' worries about their children's future, their use of and access to specialised rehabilitation services and the role of religious faith in accepting and managing the diagnosis. These two papers, published in the same year and arising from the same research programme, exemplify a complementary methodological design: the first used a standardised quality of life instrument to quantify the impact of caregiving; the second used qualitative and contextual questions to understand what that impact meant in a specific cultural setting.

9.2 The Patient Behind the Patient

Health services research has a persistent tendency to treat the patient as the exclusive unit of clinical concern. This is understandable: the patient is the person receiving treatment, and their outcomes are the stated purpose of the healthcare enterprise. But for many conditions, particularly developmental and neurodevelopmental conditions

N. Kheir, *Medicines, Patients, and the Gaps Between*,
https://doi.org/10.1007/978-981-92-5395-1_9

that require intensive, sustained and largely family-delivered management, the patient is embedded in a family system whose health and wellbeing is directly and measurably relevant to the quality of care the patient receives. Autism spectrum disorder is one of the most demanding of these conditions. It requires intensive early intervention, sustained behavioural management, navigation of specialised educational and rehabilitative services, and daily adaptation of family life to accommodate the needs of a child whose developmental trajectory is uncertain. The cumulative burden on the family caregiver, who in most Gulf contexts is the mother, operating within a cultural framework that assigns primary childcare responsibility to women, is both physiologically and psychologically significant.

By the time our research programme was designed, the international literature had already established that caregivers of children with autism experience significantly elevated rates of psychological distress, depression, anxiety and diminished physical health compared with caregivers of typically developing children and caregivers of children with other developmental disabilities. The mechanisms driving this elevated burden are multiple and interacting: the unpredictability of autistic behaviour, the social isolation that intensive caregiving imposes, the financial demands of specialised services, the strain on marital relationships and the often-inadequate support from health systems that were designed around episodic illness rather than sustained developmental care. What was almost entirely absent from this literature, at the time our studies were conducted, was evidence from Arabic-speaking and Muslim-majority societies, where the cultural frameworks shaping the caregiving experience, including the religious interpretation of disability, the role of extended family networks, the social stigma associated with neurodevelopmental conditions and the expectations placed on mothers as primary caregivers, differ substantially from those in the Western contexts that dominated the published literature.

At the time our studies were conducted (Kheir et al., 2012a; Kheir et al., 2012b), the published peer-reviewed literature contained no studies specifically examining the quality of life of caregivers of children with autism in Qatar, and the broader Arabic-speaking Middle East remained almost entirely absent from this research landscape. This was not merely a gap in the literature: it was a gap in the evidence available to policymakers planning services, to clinicians assessing families' support needs, and to the families themselves, who had no frame of reference for understanding their own experience within the local healthcare context. A further complicating factor was the demographic composition of Qatar's population: the majority of residents at the time were expatriate workers, and many families of children with autism were navigating the Qatari health and education system without the extended family networks, community supports, or linguistic resources that native Qatari families could draw upon. Designing research that was meaningful for this heterogeneous population required instruments and sampling strategies that could accommodate both Qatari nationals and expatriate residents, and an analytical sensitivity to the ways in which cultural context shaped the caregiving experience differently for different families.

9.3 What the Studies Found?

The first quality of life in autism study (Kheir et al. 2012a) recruited 98 participants: 56 caregivers of children with autism, aged 3–17 years, from the two main developmental paediatric and child rehabilitation clinics in Qatar, and 42 caregivers of typically developing children visiting a primary healthcare clinic for routine examination. Quality of life was assessed using the Lebanese Arabic version of the SF-36v2, a well-validated and widely used generic health status measure, administered by interview to protect against literacy-related bias. The findings were nuanced. Overall quality of life scores did not differ significantly between the two groups across most SF-36 domains, but caregivers of children with autism rated their health as poor and likely to worsen, a finding that was statistically significant and clinically important. Mental health scores were consistently, though not always significantly, poorer in the autism caregiver group, suggesting that the emotional toll of caregiving, while not always captured in global quality of life scores, was real and persistent.

The companion concerns and considerations study (Kheir et al. 2012b) added cultural specificity that the SF-36 could not capture. Only around 40% of caregivers in the autism group said they would encourage their child to get married and become a parent when they grew up, a finding that illustrated the depth of parental pessimism about their child's future prospects for independent adult life. Access to specialised services was a significant concern: while Qatar had made considerable investments in rehabilitation services, including speech therapy, family support groups, music therapy and sibling programmes at the clinics from which participants were recruited, many caregivers reported waiting long periods before being provided with services they needed. And religious faith emerged as a genuinely important adaptive resource: many caregivers described faith as helping them to accept the diagnosis and sustain their caregiving role, a finding consistent with the broader literature on the role of spirituality in caregiver resilience in Muslim-majority societies and one that carries direct implications for how clinical teams engage with families in the Gulf context. A clinician who fails to acknowledge the role of faith in a family's adaptive response to their child's diagnosis is missing one of the most significant psychological resources available to that family.

Taken together, the two studies painted a picture of a caregiver population that was managing considerable burden with significant resilience, but whose resilience was drawing on resources, including faith, family and community, that the formal healthcare system was largely not supporting, measuring or even acknowledging. The implication was clear: supporting these caregivers required not just better access to developmental services for their children but a deliberate, structured effort to assess and address the caregivers' own health and wellbeing as a component of the clinical care pathway.

9.4 The UREP Connection

Both publications were supported by the Qatar National Research Fund through the UREP programme, grant number UREP-06-019-3-008. This detail is more than an acknowledgement. It illustrates, in miniature, the model described in Chap. 7: undergraduate pharmacy students at Qatar University participated as active research contributors in a study that answered a genuine clinical question and produced two peer-reviewed publications in internationally recognised journals. The UREP mechanism funded the research, the students gained research experience and publication credits, and the field gained evidence it did not previously have about a patient population that had been invisible to it. This is the productive cycle that the UREP model was designed to generate, and the autism caregiver studies stand as one of its clearest illustrations.

9.5 From Research to the Classroom

The invisible patient concept that runs through this chapter became, in time, a framework that I used while teaching pharmacy practice at Qatar University and subsequently Ajman University. The argument made to students was straightforward: if you are dispensing or reviewing the medications of a child with autism, the clinical encounter you are preparing for, involves not one patient but two. The child is the pharmacological patient. The caregiver is the informational, emotional and logistical patient, the person who will administer the medications, monitor for adverse effects, manage the behavioural consequences of treatment adjustments, and return to the pharmacy with questions, concerns and sometimes significant distress. A pharmacy student who has been trained to counsel only the person in front of them at the dispensing counter will miss half of the clinical encounter that actually matters in this population.

The research findings from Kheir et al. (2012a) and Kheir et al. (2012b) were used in teaching in two ways. First, as an illustration of the measurement gap: students were asked to reflect on what the SF-36 captures and what it misses, and how the companion qualitative study revealed dimensions of the caregiving experience that the quantitative instrument could not access. This connected to the broader methodological discussion of patient-reported outcome measures that runs through the curriculum and through this book. Second, as a case study in culturally informed clinical practice: students were asked to consider how a pharmacist should respond to a caregiver who explains that they have adjusted their child's medication regimen during Ramadan, or who attributes improvement in their child's behaviour to religious practice alongside pharmacological treatment. These are not hypothetical scenarios in the Gulf context; they are the clinical realities that the research had documented, and training students to engage with them respectfully and effectively required the evidence the research had generated.

9.6 What the Field Did with These Publications?

Kheir et al. (2012a) has been cited extensively in the regional autism and caregiver quality of life literature. A study of caregiver quality of life in Oman, published in Applied Research in Quality of Life (Al-Farsi et al. 2021), cited the Qatar work as the foundational Gulf-region study against which its own findings in Omani caregivers were compared, noting that the Qatar paper had established the methodological template for caregiver quality of life assessment in the Gulf context. A 2025 scoping review of informal caregivers in the Gulf Cooperation Council region cited Kheir et al. (2012a) as a key included study, using its findings to characterise the burden profile of autism caregivers in the Gulf. A programme for Latino autistic young adults and their parents, published in a US journal in 2024, cited Kheir et al. (2012a) when arguing that caregiver support requires distinct and focused strategies tailored to the caregiver's cultural and social context. The paper has also been cited in caregiver burden studies in Ethiopia, Nigeria, Singapore and Turkey, each using the Qatar findings as a comparator data point in an international picture of caregiver quality of life.

The breadth of this citation pattern is significant. Research designed to address a gap in the Gulf context has been picked up by researchers working in Sub-Saharan Africa, Southeast Asia and North America, not because the cultural contexts are the same, but because the methodological approach of combining a validated quality of life instrument with culturally specific contextual questions provided a replicable template for caregiver research in any setting where the dominant literature does not adequately reflect local conditions. The research contributed to the field's methodological vocabulary as much as to its substantive findings.

9.7 The Pharmacy's Missing Role

What strikes me, in retrospect, about both studies is how completely the pharmacy was absent from the caregiving picture they described. Families managing a child with autism in Qatar were navigating a complex landscape of medical appointments, behavioural interventions, educational placements, and, in many cases, medication management. Psychotropic medications are commonly used in autism management to address associated behaviours, including sleep disturbances, anxiety and self-injurious behaviour, and the medication management burden in this population, particularly for families with limited health literacy or language barriers, is real and largely unaddressed by the pharmacy profession in the Gulf. There is no published literature on pharmacist involvement in the medication management of children with autism in Qatar, or indeed in most MENA countries. That absence is not a reflection of the profession's lack of capacity. It is a reflection of the absence of a professional mandate and a structured service model for pharmacist involvement in this population.

The caregivers who participated in our quality of life in parents of children with autism studies were managing medication regimens, monitoring behavioural responses to treatment, and navigating a fragmented healthcare system, all without any structured pharmacist input. The treatment burden concept developed in Chap. 2 of this book is directly applicable to this population: the administrative, logistical, and cognitive demands of managing a child's complex medication regimen, across multiple prescribers and multiple specialties, constitutes a measurable and modifiable burden that pharmacist-led medication review is well positioned to address. That that positioning was not recognised or acted upon in the years following these studies is one of the clearest examples in this book of the gap between what pharmaceutical care promises and what the caregiving population actually received.

9.8 The Gap the Research Left Open

Both studies were cross-sectional, capturing the caregiving experience at a single point in time. The quality of life of caregivers of children with autism is not static: it changes with the child's developmental progress, with the availability and quality of services, with the caregiver's own health trajectory, and with the social and financial circumstances of the family over time. Longitudinal studies would have told a more complete story about which caregivers are most vulnerable to sustained quality of life deterioration and what factors either accelerate or protect against that deterioration. Those studies have not been conducted in the Gulf context.

A second gap is the exclusive focus on mothers as the primary caregiver unit. In the Gulf context, the extended family network, including fathers, grandparents and siblings, plays a significant role in the daily management of a child with autism, and the burden experienced by these non-primary caregivers has not been examined. In a family system where the father's role in navigating institutional relationships, financial management and religious interpretation of disability is distinct from the mother's role in daily care, a research programme that studies only mothers is capturing only part of the caregiving system. The policy and service implications of a fuller picture of the whole family's experience could be substantial.

A third gap is the absence of any intervention component. Both studies documented burden and identified its correlates, but neither tested whether any pharmacist-delivered, clinician-delivered or service-level intervention could reduce that burden or improve caregiver quality of life. The measurement without action gap, identified as one of the three structural themes of this book in the Introduction, is nowhere more apparent than here: a population whose burden was documented with precision in 2012 has still not been the subject of a single intervention study targeting caregiver wellbeing in the Qatari or Gulf context.

9.9 Research Agenda Note

The caregiver research programme documented in this chapter points toward five open questions that remain unanswered and that represent the most important unfinished work in this area for the Gulf context.

First: what is the longitudinal trajectory of quality of life among caregivers of children with autism in Gulf societies, and which child, caregiver and service-level factors predict sustained deterioration versus resilience over a 5-year horizon? A prospective cohort study following the caregivers documented in our first study (study a) or a new cohort recruited from the same clinical settings would address the most fundamental limitation of the cross-sectional design.

Second: can a structured pharmacist-led medication management service for caregivers of children with autism, involving regular medication review, caregiver education about psychotropic medications and their monitoring, and active coordination with the treating clinical team, reduce medication-related burden and improve caregiver quality of life? The treatment burden framework developed in Chap. 2 provides the theoretical foundation for such a service, and the absence of any pharmacist involvement documented in this chapter provides the clinical justification for testing it.

Third: what is the prevalence and character of medication-related burden among caregivers managing psychotropic and other medications for children with autism in Gulf primary care and specialist settings, and how does that burden relate to caregiver quality of life and to child clinical outcomes? This is a measurement question that precedes the intervention question but that has not yet been asked in the Gulf context.

Fourth: how do the caregiving experiences and quality of life of fathers, grandparents and extended family members in Gulf autism families differ from those of mothers, and what does that difference imply for the design of family-centred clinical support services and carer education programmes? Answering this question requires both quantitative comparison of quality of life across caregiver roles and qualitative exploration of the different ways in which extended family members understand and manage their caregiving responsibilities.

Fifth: can the integration of a validated caregiver quality of life assessment tool into the routine clinical care pathway for autism services in Gulf health systems improve the identification of caregivers at risk of health deterioration and increase referrals to appropriate psychosocial and practical support? This is an implementation research question that tests whether measurement alone, when embedded in clinical workflow, changes clinical behaviour and improves caregiver outcomes.

9.10 What Remains?

Caregiver health is a legitimate healthcare outcome and its systematic assessment is a legitimate healthcare responsibility. The two publications documented in this chapter made a genuine contribution to establishing that principle in the Qatari context, providing the first evidence base for caregiver quality of life in Gulf autism families and generating a methodological template that subsequent researchers in the region and beyond have drawn on. What they could not do was change the practice environment in which those caregivers were operating. More than a decade after these studies were published, the pharmacy profession in the Gulf has still not developed a structured role in the medication management of children with autism or in the support of their caregivers. The research agenda points clearly toward the next steps. Whether those steps are taken depends on whether the profession, the health system, and the funding bodies that support research in this region choose to treat the family behind the patient as a legitimate clinical concern rather than a background variable.[1]

References

Al-Farsi YM, Al-Sharbati MM, Al-Farsi O, Al-Shafaee M, Brooks DR, Waly MI (2021) Quality of life among caregivers of children with autism spectrum disorders, intellectual disability, and typical development. Appl Res Qual Life 16:939–953

Kheir N, Ghoneim O, Sandridge AL, Al-Ismail M, Hayder S, Al-Rawi F (2012a) Quality of life of caregivers of children with autism in Qatar. Autism 16(3):293–298*

Kheir NM, Ghoneim OM, Sandridge AL, Hayder SA, Al-Ismail MS, Al-Rawi F (2012b) Concerns and considerations among caregivers of a child with autism in Qatar. BMC Res Notes 5:290*

[1]Publications by the author of this book are marked with an asterisk (*) in references.

Chapter 10
Tobacco, Warnings and the Limits of Persuasion

10.1 The Anchor Publication

This chapter is built around Awaisu et al. (2013), published in Nicotine and Tobacco Research, which evaluated the general public's awareness, beliefs, and perceptions of anti-tobacco pictorial health warning labels on cigarette packs prior to the implementation of new pictorial warning legislation in Qatar. The study was conducted at Qatar University's College of Pharmacy, and the author of this book was one of four co-investigators on the research team. The paper addressed a specific and practically important question: before pictorial warnings were mandated and introduced on tobacco packaging in Qatar, what did the public know about them, what did they believe about their effectiveness and what could that pre-implementation baseline tell policymakers about what to expect when the new warnings arrived?

10.2 The Tobacco Burden in Qatar

Tobacco use in Qatar is a public health problem of considerable magnitude. At the time the study was conducted, estimates placed adult male smoking prevalence in Qatar at between 37% and 40%, and conservative calculations suggested that at least one billion cigarettes were smoked in Qatar each year, generating approximately US$150 million in annual healthcare expenditure related to tobacco-caused illness (Awaisu et al. 2013). The Qatar population's particular demographic character, predominantly young, predominantly male and predominantly expatriate, created a tobacco use landscape that was both epidemiologically significant and culturally specific: patterns of tobacco product use that extended well beyond cigarettes to include waterpipe tobacco, which was socially normalised and substantially under-regulated, and to smokeless tobacco products that existed at the margins of regulatory attention.

N. Kheir, *Medicines, Patients, and the Gaps Between*,
https://doi.org/10.1007/978-981-92-5395-1_10

The adoption of pictorial health warnings represented Qatar's alignment with the WHO Framework Convention on Tobacco Control (FCTC), which it had ratified, and with the growing international evidence that graphic, emotionally evocative warnings on tobacco packaging were more effective than text-only warnings at increasing awareness of health risks, stimulating cessation intentions and reducing tobacco consumption, particularly among younger smokers and those with lower health literacy. The FCTC, adopted in 2003 and ratified by more than 180 countries, represented the first global health treaty negotiated under the auspices of the World Health Organization. Article 11 of the Convention requires that tobacco product packaging carry health warnings that are large, clear, visible and legible, and recommends that these include pictures or pictograms. Qatar's move toward pictorial warnings was therefore both a public health decision and an international treaty obligation, and the pre-implementation study was designed to provide the evidence base that responsible implementation required.

10.3 The International Evidence on Pictorial Warnings

The scientific case for pictorial health warnings had been building for more than a decade before the Qatar study was conducted. Canada introduced graphic warning labels in 2001, becoming the first country to mandate pictorial warnings on cigarette packaging, and the evidence from the Canadian experience established a template that other countries and researchers would follow: warnings increased health knowledge, increased cessation calls to telephone quit lines, and were associated with reduced smoking prevalence, particularly among younger smokers. Brazil, Australia, Thailand and numerous other countries followed with their own mandatory pictorial warning regimes, each generating evaluation data that the international research community synthesised into an increasingly robust evidence base.

By the time Awaisu et al. (2013) was published, the international literature had established several consistent findings. Pictorial warnings are more effective than text-only warnings across multiple outcomes, including awareness of health risks, emotional response, cessation intentions and cessation attempts. Larger warnings are more effective than smaller ones, which provided the regulatory rationale for the progressive increase in required warning size that most FCTC signatories implemented over successive regulatory cycles. Warnings depicting vivid, emotionally evocative health consequences, including diseased lungs, mouth cancer and children affected by secondhand smoke, are more effective than abstract or diagrammatic warnings. And warnings are most effective when combined with cessation support resources, including quit lines, nicotine replacement therapy and pharmacist-delivered cessation counselling, because the warning can stimulate a cessation intention that the healthcare system then needs the capacity to support. This last finding was the one most consistently overlooked in Qatar's regulatory environment, and it is the finding that this chapter returns to in reflecting on what the research left unaddressed.

10.4 What the Pre-Implementation Study Found?

The study administered a 23-item pre-tested questionnaire to 500 randomly approached adults in Qatar, representing the demographic diversity of the resident population, and the findings were sobering in ways that the policymakers introducing the new legislation needed to understand before implementation rather than after. Approximately one-third of respondents had no knowledge of any specific text warning message currently on tobacco products sold in Qatar, and nearly 45% did not know what a pictorial health warning was (Awaisu et al. 2013). Crucially, ever-smokers did not differ significantly from never-smokers in their awareness of pictorial warnings, a finding that undermined a common assumption, that tobacco users are already well-informed about health risks and that warnings primarily reach non-users, and suggested that both groups would be arriving at the pictorial warning experience with similarly limited contextual knowledge.

More than 20% of respondents in both smoker and non-smoker groups did not believe that introducing pictorial warnings would enhance smoking behaviour change, a finding that pointed to a pre-existing scepticism about regulatory persuasion that the implementation programme would need to address. Non-smokers generally held more positive attitudes than smokers toward the perceived impact of warnings, a pattern consistent with the international literature and with the psychological principle that individuals with a personal stake in maintaining a behaviour are more likely to engage in motivated reasoning that discounts the evidence against it. The study also found that younger respondents and those with higher educational attainment were more aware of pictorial warnings and more supportive of their implementation, a pattern with direct implications for the design of complementary communication campaigns targeting older smokers and those with lower literacy levels, who would be least likely to respond to the warnings without additional support.

10.5 From Research to the Classroom

The tobacco control research documented in this chapter connected to pharmacy education in ways that were both direct and generative. At Qatar University's College of Pharmacy, the findings of Awaisu et al. (2013) were used in teaching health promotion and patient counselling, as a case study in the distinction between awareness, attitude and behaviour. Students were presented with the finding that nearly half of respondents did not know what a pictorial warning was, and asked what role the community pharmacist could play in bridging that awareness gap at the point of sale. The discussion that followed consistently surfaced a tension that runs through pharmacy education in the Gulf: students understood conceptually what the pharmacist's role in tobacco cessation could and should be, but they had limited exposure to the structured counselling skills and behaviour change frameworks that would allow them to fulfil that role in practice.

This gap became a teaching case for the Transtheoretical Model of Change described in Chap. 2 of this book. A smoker who has just read a pictorial warning depicting diseased lungs and has experienced, perhaps for the first time, a genuine intention to quit, is in the contemplation or preparation stage of change. A pharmacist trained only to dispense nicotine replacement therapy, without the skills to assess the smoker's stage of change, explore their barriers to cessation and provide stage-matched counselling, will miss the clinical window that the warning has opened. Teaching students to connect the public health intervention of the warning label to the individual clinical intervention of the pharmacy consultation was one of the most practically useful things the tobacco research made possible in the educational context.

10.6 What the Field Did with This Publication?

Awaisu et al. (2013) entered a literature that was actively building the evidence base for pictorial warning policy in the Gulf and broader developing world context, and it contributed to that literature at a specific and useful moment: the pre-implementation phase, which provided a baseline against which post-implementation changes could eventually be measured. The paper was cited in a Saudi Dental Journal review of tobacco control accomplishments and challenges across the Gulf Cooperation Council countries, which used it as one of the few peer-reviewed data points on the Qatari tobacco control landscape. It was cited in studies of pictorial warning effectiveness in Jordan, in waterpipe-specific warning research among university students, and in studies from Nepal, Indonesia and Mauritius, where researchers used the Qatar pre-implementation data to contextualise their own findings on the trajectory of awareness and attitudes before and after mandatory warning introduction. The paper was also cited in a systematic review of pictorial cigarette pack warnings published in the American Journal of Public Health (Monarrez-Espino et al. 2014), which included it as one of the regional studies contributing to the global evidence base on warning effectiveness.

The international reach of the citations is noteworthy for the same reason noted in Chap. 9: a study designed for a specific Gulf policy context was picked up by researchers across Southeast Asia, South Asia and the African continent. The methodological contribution, a pre-implementation design with a demographically representative sampling strategy in a FCTC signatory country with high expatriate population density, provided a replicable template that other countries facing similar implementation decisions found useful. The research functioned simultaneously as local policy evidence and as a contribution to the global methodology of tobacco warning evaluation.

10.7 The Limits of Persuasion

The honest reflection that this research invites is about the limits of persuasion as a public health strategy, and about what pictorial warnings can and cannot do. The international evidence, consistently replicated across settings and time periods, supports the conclusion that pictorial warnings increase awareness of health risks and raise cessation intentions, particularly among younger smokers and those less committed to continuing. These are real effects, and they are worth having. But the distance between increased cessation intention and actual cessation behaviour is, as every clinician working in tobacco cessation knows, considerable, and it is bridged primarily by the availability, quality and accessibility of cessation support, not by the warning label alone.

In Qatar, as in most of the Gulf, the pharmacist's role in cessation support remains substantially underdeveloped. Community pharmacies are among the most accessible points of contact in the healthcare system for the tobacco-using population, many of whom do not have a regular primary care physician and who may use the community pharmacy as their primary point of access to health information and over-the-counter medications. The pharmacist in that setting is uniquely positioned to initiate a brief intervention conversation, to assess readiness to quit, to recommend or supply nicotine replacement therapy, and to refer patients to structured cessation programmes. The policy investment in pictorial warnings, well-grounded in the evidence, has not been matched by an equivalent investment in the cessation support infrastructure that would allow smokers who respond to those warnings to act on their intentions. That mismatch is one of the clearest examples in this book of the evidence-practice gap: a population-level intervention producing an intention that the healthcare system is insufficiently equipped to convert into behaviour change.

10.8 The Gap the Research Left Open

The pre-implementation study established a baseline. The natural scientific successor to a pre-implementation study is a post-implementation study, using the same methodology and the same population, to measure whether the introduction of pictorial warnings changed awareness, attitudes and, ultimately, smoking behaviour. That follow-up study, to the best of our knowledge, has not been published from Qatar. Without it, the pre-implementation data remain informative but incomplete: a baseline without the longitudinal comparison that would allow its policy implications to be fully evaluated. This is not a critique of the original study, which was well designed for its stated purpose. It is an acknowledgement of the research gap that a pre-implementation study always implies and that post-implementation studies must eventually fill.

A second gap is the near-complete absence of waterpipe tobacco from the research agenda. The Awaisu et al. (2013) study focused on cigarette packaging warnings, reflecting the regulatory focus of the period. Waterpipe tobacco, however, is a distinct product with a distinct cultural status in Gulf societies, a distinct pattern of use, and a distinct population of users, many of whom do not identify as smokers and who are therefore unlikely to be reached by cigarette-focused warning campaigns. The evidence on waterpipe-specific warnings was, at the time of the original study, thin globally and almost non-existent in the Gulf context. It remains underrepresented in the regional tobacco control literature relative to the scale of waterpipe use and the evidence of its health consequences.

10.9 Research Agenda Note

The tobacco control research programme documented in this chapter points toward five open questions that represent the most important unfinished work in this area for the Gulf context.

First: what changes in awareness, attitudes and tobacco use behaviour occurred in Qatar's resident population following the implementation of pictorial health warnings on tobacco packaging, and how do those changes compare with the pre-implementation baseline established by Awaisu et al. (2013)? A post-implementation study using the same sampling strategy and the same questionnaire items would answer the most fundamental unanswered question the original study raised, and it is a study that can still be conducted.

Second: what is the comparative effectiveness of pictorial health warnings specifically designed for waterpipe tobacco products in reducing waterpipe tobacco use in Qatar and the wider Gulf, and which warning design features, images, sizes and placement, are most effective in the Gulf cultural context where waterpipe use carries distinct social meanings that cigarette-focused warnings do not address?

Third: can a structured pharmacist-delivered brief intervention programme for tobacco cessation, using established behaviour change frameworks, incorporating nicotine replacement therapy supply and adapted for the linguistic and cultural diversity of Qatar's population, reduce smoking rates among adult tobacco users presenting at community pharmacies? This is a randomised controlled trial question, and the community pharmacy infrastructure in Qatar, with its high density of trained pharmacists and its accessibility to the tobacco-using population, provides a realistic setting in which to test it.

Fourth: how do awareness of and attitudinal responses to pictorial health warnings differ across the major expatriate communities in Qatar, and what does that variation imply for the design of multilingual and culturally adapted tobacco control communication strategies that reach beyond the Arabic and English-speaking populations targeted by current warning designs?

Fifth: what is the impact of formally integrating tobacco cessation counselling as a structured, remunerated component of community pharmacy practice in Qatar on cessation rates, on pharmacist professional satisfaction and on healthcare system costs relative to the current standard of care? This is an implementation research and health economics question, and answering it would provide the evidence base that pharmacy professional bodies and health ministries need to justify the regulatory and financial investment in pharmacist-delivered cessation services.

10.10 What Remains?

The tobacco control agenda in Qatar and the wider Gulf is unfinished in ways that are specific to the regional context. Waterpipe tobacco remains substantially under-regulated compared with cigarettes, despite evidence that its health risks are comparable, and despite the particular social normalisation of waterpipe use in Gulf societies that makes regulatory intervention both more necessary and more politically complicated. The demographic diversity of Qatar's resident population creates health communication challenges that warnings in Arabic and English alone cannot fully address. And the pharmacist's potential role in cessation support, well-documented in the international literature and clearly implied by the research documented in this chapter, has not been systematically developed, evaluated or institutionalised in the Gulf context. The evidence base on pictorial warnings justified the policy. Closing the gap between warning and cessation requires a different kind of investment, in accessible, pharmacist-delivered, culturally adapted cessation support, and that investment has not yet been made at the scale the burden of tobacco use in the Gulf demands.[1]

References

Awaisu A, Hagi A, Ashour MA, Kheir N (2013) Pictorial health warnings on cigarette packages in Qatar: preimplementation awareness and perceptions of ever-smokers versus never-smokers. Nicotine Tob Res 15(10):1765–1772*

Monárrez-Espino J, Liu B, Greiner F, Bremberg S, Galanti R (2014) Systematic review of the effect of pictorial warnings on cigarette packages in smoking behavior. Am J Public Health 104(10):e11–e30

[1]Publications by the author of this book are marked with an asterisk (*) in references.

Chapter 11
COVID-19 and Medicines Access: A Stress Test for Systems and Assumptions

11.1 The Anchor Publication

This chapter is built around Kheir et al. (2023), published as a living reference work entry in the Springer Encyclopedia of Evidence in Pharmaceutical Public Health and Health Services Research in Pharmacy (DOI: 10.1007/978-3-030-50247-8_108-1). The entry was submitted in July 2021, accepted in May 2022, and published online in February 2023. It documented and synthesised the disruptions to medicines access that the COVID-19 pandemic created globally, covering supply chain fragility, differential impacts on low- and middle-income countries, access to vaccines, pharmaceutical access for acute and chronic conditions, the expanded role of community pharmacy and a set of challenges, opportunities and recommendations for patients, health professionals and policymakers. As an encyclopaedia entry, this publication occupies a different genre from the empirical studies that anchor most other chapters in this book. It is a synthesising work rather than a primary research study, and its contribution is evaluative and documentary rather than experimental. That difference in genre requires a correspondingly different kind of retrospective analysis: rather than asking what the study found and what the field did with it, this chapter asks what the encyclopaedia entry contributed to the scholarly record, what it could and could not say given its genre and what the events it documented have since revealed about the structural vulnerabilities of medicines access systems globally.

11.2 The Pandemic as a Natural Experiment

Public health researchers sometimes speak of natural experiments: events that create the conditions for studying questions that would be impossible or unethical to design experimentally. The COVID-19 pandemic was a natural experiment of extraordinary,

N. Kheir, *Medicines, Patients, and the Gaps Between*,
https://doi.org/10.1007/978-981-92-5395-1_11

if devastating, scale. In the space of weeks, it disrupted every aspect of the global healthcare system, including the medicines supply chain, the functioning of community and hospital pharmacies, the management of chronic conditions whose routine care was deferred or interrupted and the medication access patterns of populations who found their normal healthcare pathways blocked or overwhelmed. These disruptions were not uniform: they fell differently on different countries, different patient populations, different disease groups and different health system structures, and the pattern of those differences was itself revealing about the structural vulnerabilities that had been present before the pandemic but had not been stress-tested at this scale.

The encyclopaedia entry documented the scale of these disruptions with specificity. More than 30 pharmaceutical factories in China that manufacture active pharmaceutical ingredients for drug companies in the United States were closed in response to the pandemic (Kheir et al. 2023). India, the world's largest producer of generic drugs, began experiencing delays in receiving active ingredients from China and could not keep up with global demand. In a 6-month period in 2020, drug shortages reached the equivalent of 87% of the total shortages reported for the entire year of 2019 (Kheir et al. 2023). These figures were not aberrations. They were the predictable consequence of a supply chain architecture that had prioritised efficiency over resilience, concentrating production in a small number of countries without building the redundancy that a global health emergency would require. The entry identified this structural fragility as the most acutely exposed pre-existing vulnerability: the pandemic had not created it; it had revealed it, suddenly and at scale.

The differential impact on low- and middle-income countries was pronounced. In Nigeria, a study reported that approximately 35% of patients with chronic illnesses had difficulties accessing essential medicines during the COVID-19 lockdown, with around 84% experiencing deteriorating chronic health conditions as a direct result (Kheir et al. 2023). Over 75% of patients with chronic health conditions in that study could not afford medicines, and around 80% reported that their income had been negatively affected by the pandemic. Alongside these access failures, the global vaccine equity gap was equally stark: by mid-May 2021, only 0.3% of total doses of approved vaccines had been distributed to low-income countries (Kheir et al. 2023), a figure that illustrated the distance between the international community's stated commitments to equitable access and the reality of who received what, and when.

11.3 What the Pandemic Revealed About Pharmacy?

For pharmacy specifically, the pandemic created both a crisis and an opportunity, and the balance between them differed substantially across health system contexts. In the crisis register, pharmacies faced increased demand for medications, staff illness and workforce disruption, supply unpredictability that made inventory management genuinely difficult and the need to implement infection control measures that changed the physical environment of patient interaction in ways that were simultaneously necessary and clinically suboptimal. Community pharmacies in many settings, operating on thin margins with minimal redundancy in staffing or stock, were stressed in ways that the health system had not anticipated because pharmacy had not been integrated into pandemic preparedness planning in ways commensurate with its essential health service function.

In the opportunity register, the pandemic demonstrated, more visibly than any previous event in recent memory, that pharmacists were essential health workers capable of adapting rapidly to changed circumstances. The encyclopaedia entry documented that community pharmacists in progressive pharmacy practice settings took on medication management services, infectious disease mitigation, point-of-care testing, and vaccination administration; that home delivery services were mobilised to reach patients who could not attend pharmacies in person; and that the pandemic drew renewed attention to the decades-long argument from pharmacy leaders, regulators and academics for the wide adoption of patient-centred pharmaceutical care services (Kheir et al. 2023). In many countries, the pandemic expanded the scope of pharmacist practice by necessity, in ways that regulatory frameworks had previously resisted. Whether those expansions have been retained as permanent features of pharmacy practice, or whether they have been quietly withdrawn as the acute emergency receded, is a country-by-country question that the literature is only beginning to answer.

11.4 The Gulf Context

The Gulf states, including Qatar and the UAE, occupied a specific position in the global COVID-19 medicines access landscape that the encyclopaedia entry's global synthesis could only partially capture. As high-income countries with relatively well-resourced health systems, they were less exposed than low- and middle-income countries to the most severe medicines access disruptions of the pandemic. But their high dependence on imported pharmaceuticals, their large expatriate populations with heterogeneous health profiles and varying access to formal healthcare, and their reliance on global supply chains for both finished pharmaceutical products and active pharmaceutical ingredients, created vulnerabilities that the pandemic exposed with unusual clarity.

Both Qatar and the UAE responded with notable speed at the pharmacy and health system level. Qatar's Primary Health Care Corporation launched a home medication delivery service for chronic disease patients, elderly residents and pregnant women in March 2020, and virtual consultations reached approximately 50% of total consultation volumes within weeks of the pandemic's onset. The UAE's response was equally proactive: safe working practice guidelines for community pharmacies were issued in late March 2020, the Abu Dhabi Department of Health published pharmacy medication delivery standards before the WHO global pandemic declaration, and digital medicines access through the nationally available 800 pharmacy application was rapidly mobilised during lockdown periods. A hospital pharmacy study from Al Ain Hospital documented pharmaceutical adaptations during the acute phase and reported high levels of patient and physician satisfaction with services including home medication delivery and remote clinical pharmacy support (Hammad et al. 2023). Despite these commendable system-level responses, detailed peer-reviewed documentation of medicines access outcomes across the Gulf during the pandemic remains sparse, representing a missed opportunity for health systems learning.

The migrant worker dimension of medicines access in the Gulf during COVID-19 also deserves specific attention. Qatar's population at the time of the pandemic was predominantly non-national, with a large proportion of workers in low-wage employment whose access to formal healthcare, including prescription medicines, was structurally constrained by employment conditions, insurance coverage gaps, language barriers, and in some cases fear of detection or deportation. The global literature on COVID-19 and health inequity consistently identified migrant and mobile populations as among those most severely affected by medicines access disruptions (Kheir et al. 2023). The Gulf's specific configuration of this problem, large numbers of workers in concentrated accommodation with limited access to community pharmacy, prescription medicines or chronic disease management, was a regional manifestation of a global pattern that the encyclopaedia entry documented at a general level without the regional specificity that the Gulf context required.

11.5 From Research to the Classroom

The encyclopaedia entry was written during a period of faculty exchange from Ajman University to the University of Auckland, in collaboration with colleague academics from the School of Pharmacy at Auckland: Amy Chan, Shane Scahill and Kebede Beyene. That collaborative context was directly relevant to the intellectual substance of what was written. New Zealand's pharmacy system, relatively progressive in its recognition of extended pharmacist roles and its integration of community pharmacy into primary healthcare, provided a counterpoint to the Gulf systems the author knew best, and the Auckland colleagues' firsthand experience of pharmacy practice during the New Zealand COVID-19 response informed the sections on pharmacist role expansion, home delivery services and scope of practice debates in ways that a geographically isolated author could not have achieved.

The experience of writing this entry during a period when the pandemic was still unfolding gave it a pedagogical character that a retrospective synthesis would not have had. The questions it was trying to answer, about supply chain vulnerability, vaccine equity, the pharmacist's essential worker status and the ethics of medicines access in crisis conditions, were not settled questions with established answers. They were live questions being debated in real time, and the process of assembling the evidence, identifying what was known and what remained unknown, and formulating recommendations for policymakers under conditions of genuine uncertainty was itself a model of the kind of evidence-informed reasoning that pharmacy education should be cultivating. Whether or not that connection was made explicit in the classroom at the time, it represents one of the clearest examples in this book of research and scholarship emerging from, and speaking back to, the professional world the researcher inhabits.

11.6 What the Field Did with This Publication?

Encyclopaedia entries occupy a specific and somewhat unusual position in the scholarly citation economy. They are cited as reference works rather than as primary evidence, and they are typically consulted by readers seeking orientation to a field rather than by specialists seeking to engage with specific findings. The Kheir et al. (2023) entry has been cited in subsequent public health literature on medicines access during health system crises, in teaching materials on pharmaceutical systems and global health, and in policy-oriented documents that used the encyclopaedia as a source of documentary synthesis on the pandemic's pharmaceutical impact. Its contribution is primarily informational and organisational: it assembled and ordered knowledge that was otherwise scattered across a rapidly expanding pandemic literature, making it accessible to readers who needed a structured overview rather than primary research.

11.7 The Gap the Research Left Open

The encyclopaedia entry format is inherently constrained in what it can argue and how directly it can argue it. Its genre requires synthesis and documentation rather than critique and advocacy, and its audience is general rather than specialist. The medicines access disruptions it documented raised questions that the entry format could note but not pursue: questions about why supply chain concentration had been permitted to reach the levels of fragility that the pandemic exposed, about who bore the greatest burden of medicines access disruption and why, about what policy changes were required to prevent the recurrence of the same vulnerabilities and about whether the pharmacy profession's expanded role during the pandemic would be institutionalised or abandoned once the emergency passed. Pursuing those questions would have required a different kind of publication: a commentary, a policy analysis or a research paper with a specific empirical question. That the encyclopaedia entry did not take on those questions is a function of its genre not a failure of its authors. But the questions remain and the research agenda they imply is not one that the encyclopaedia entry itself can complete.

11.8 Research Agenda Note

The medicines access research documented in this chapter points toward five open questions that the encyclopaedia entry raised but could not answer.

First: what was the actual impact of COVID-19 on medicines access for patients with non-communicable diseases in health systems in the Middle East and globally, measured in terms of medication discontinuation rates, chronic disease exacerbation and patient-reported outcomes? The global literature on this question is growing but the Gulf-specific evidence base remains thin, and the regional health systems that managed the pandemic with relative effectiveness have not yet produced the detailed documentation of their pharmaceutical system performance that would allow others to learn from their experience.

Second: have the expanded pharmacy scopes of practice implemented during the COVID-19 pandemic been formally retained in regulatory frameworks, and what evidence exists that these expansions improved patient outcomes during the emergency period? Answering this question requires both regulatory analysis and outcomes data, and it matters because the case for permanent scope expansion depends on demonstrating that the expanded practice was safe, effective and valued by patients.

Third: what structural changes to pharmaceutical supply chain management and strategic stockpiling have health ministries implemented since the COVID-19 pandemic, and are those changes sufficient to prevent comparable medicines access disruptions during future health emergencies of similar or greater scale? This is a policy analysis question that requires engagement with health ministry data and regulatory documentation that the peer-reviewed literature has not yet systematically assembled.

Fourth: how did the COVID-19 pandemic differentially affect medicines access specifically for the Gulf states, known for their large migrant worker populations compared with national residents, and what does that differential tell us about the structural determinants of medicines access equity in high-income states with high proportions of non-citizen residents? This is both an equity research question and a human rights question, and it has significant implications for the design of emergency preparedness systems that are genuinely inclusive of all residents rather than primarily designed around the needs of citizens.

Fifth: what role did community pharmacists actually play in maintaining medicines access and providing patient care in health systems during the acute phase of the COVID-19 pandemic, and has that contribution been formally documented, recognised, and incorporated into subsequent emergency preparedness planning at the national levels? The absence of documentation of pharmacy's pandemic contribution is itself a finding about the profession's institutional visibility and its integration into health system governance.

11.9 What Remains?

The medicines access disruptions of the COVID-19 pandemic have not been resolved by the pandemic's transition to endemic status. Supply chain concentration has been acknowledged as a strategic vulnerability by governments and international organisations, but the structural changes required to meaningfully address it, including diversification of active pharmaceutical ingredient production, strategic stockpiling, and international coordination frameworks for essential medicines security, are politically complex and commercially costly, and they have advanced more slowly than the urgency of the pandemic period suggested they would. The inequities in medicines access between high-income and low- and middle-income countries that the pandemic exposed were not created by COVID-19 and have not been remedied by its passage. And pharmacy's role as an essential health service, demonstrated with unusual clarity during the pandemic, remains formally unrecognised in emergency preparedness frameworks in most health systems, including those of the Gulf and wider Middle East. The pandemic was a demonstration of what the evidence on medicines access had been suggesting for years: that the systems through which people obtain the medicines they need are more fragile, more inequitable and more dependent on the resilience of frontline health workers than most health system planners had assumed. That demonstration was costly. Acting on what it revealed has been slower.[1]

References

Hammad M, Tashtoush MM, El Faki EMA, Hajaj MY, Ahmed SS, Darwish AA (2023) Hospital pharmacy response to the COVID-19 pandemic: experience from a regional referral center in the United Arab Emirates. J Pharm Policy Pract 16:36

Kheir N, Chan A, Scahill S, Beyene K (2023) COVID-19 and medicines access. In: Babar ZUD (ed) Encyclopedia of evidence in pharmaceutical public health and health services research in pharmacy. Springer, Cham*

[1]Publications by the author of this book are marked with an asterisk (*) in references.

Chapter 12
What the Research Taught the Researcher: A Closing Reflection

The Introduction to this book proposed that the gap between what pharmacy promises and what patients receive manifests in three related but distinct themes across the chapters: the evidence-practice gap, the education-environment gap and the measurement-action gap. Returning to that framework at the close, having examined twelve research programmes in detail, it is worth assessing whether the framework held up under examination and what it reveals that a chapter-by-chapter reading alone might not.

The evidence-practice gap proved the most documented and the least resolved. From the pharmaceutical care framework studies of Chap. 1 to the counselling audit of Chap. 5 to the adherence barrier research of Chap. 8 and the tobacco warning pre-implementation study of Chap. 10, the same finding recurred in different settings, with different patient populations, and using different methodologies: pharmacy practitioners consistently fell short of the evidence-based standard that the profession had articulated as its aspiration. What the research programme documented with increasing precision over two decades was not a moving target but a stable one: the evidence-practice gap in pharmacy in the Arab Middle East did not close over the period this book covers. It was confirmed, refined and contextualised but not closed. That is an uncomfortable finding and a necessary one.

The education-environment gap proved the most theoretically generative. The disconnect between the quality of graduates produced by well-designed pharmacy programmes and the quality of professional practice they delivered in their working environments pointed, more clearly than any other theme in this book, to the inadequacy of individual-level explanations of professional behaviour. A graduate cannot sustain pharmaceutical care practice in an environment that does not support, expect or remunerate it, regardless of how well they were trained. That insight has implications beyond pharmacy education: it argues for a fundamentally systems-level conception of professional practice development, one that attends as seriously to the regulatory, economic and cultural conditions of practice as it does to the knowledge and skills of individual practitioners. Chapter Six provided the most concentrated illustration of

N. Kheir, *Medicines, Patients, and the Gaps Between*,
https://doi.org/10.1007/978-981-92-5395-1_12

this, but it ran as a current through Chaps. 1, 5 and 7, and it connects the pharmacy education research to the broader literature on professional identity formation and workplace learning that the field has increasingly engaged with.

The measurement-action gap proved the most morally significant. Documenting the quality of life burden of caregivers of children with autism in Qatar (Chap. 9), or the medication-related burden of patients with chronic kidney disease in primary care (Chap. 2), or the adherence barriers experienced by patients with uncontrolled diabetes (Chap. 8), without subsequently investigating whether any pharmacist-delivered intervention could address what was measured, is a form of research incompleteness that carries a cost. The patients and caregivers who participated in those studies did so in the understanding that their participation would contribute to better care. Research that measures without acting, that describes without testing, that publishes without following up, has partially but not fully honoured that understanding. This is not a counsel of guilt; it is an argument for sequencing research programmes more deliberately, so that measurement studies generate intervention studies rather than simply generating citation counts.

12.1 The Full Circle, Examined Honestly

This book has attempted to demonstrate, across eleven substantive chapters, that the full circle between research and practice is achievable, but that it requires more than publishing the findings. The citation trails documented in each chapter are evidence that translation occurs, unevenly, slowly, and often in unexpected directions, but it does occur. Kheir et al. (2001) found its way into a 2018 global meta-analysis (Dokbua et al. 2018) and into Iraqi pharmacy education research in 2025 (Yassen et al. 2025). Kheir et al. (2008) became the baseline reference for a field and was still being cited and updated nearly two decades after its publication. Zidan et al. (2016a) generated the subsequent quasi-experimental study by El Hajj et al. (2023) that provided the outcomes evidence the protocol had been designed to enable. Jaam et al. (2018a) was cited in a 2025 Qatari study that built on its findings to examine service delivery gaps in diabetes management. Kheir et al. (2012a) reached caregivers of autistic young adults in the United States, where researchers cited it to argue that caregiver support requires culturally adapted strategies. These are real contributions, and they deserve to be named as such.

But the full circle, examined honestly, is rarely as clean as a citation trail makes it appear. A citation does not prove that practice changed. It proves that a subsequent researcher found the work worth referencing, which is a necessary but insufficient condition for impact. The deeper question, whether the patients whose circumstances the research described received better care because the research was done, is a question that the peer-reviewed literature rarely answers directly, and that the research programmes documented in this book answer only partially and imperfectly. The medication-related burden framework was measured but not systematically acted on in clinical practice. The counselling gap was precisely documented and then mostly confirmed by subsequent studies rather than closed by subsequent interventions. The pharmaceutical care reform was advanced in curricula and stalled in community pharmacies. The tobacco warning research established a baseline that has not yet been followed by the post-implementation comparison it implied. These are honest assessments, and a book that claimed otherwise would be a different kind of book: one less useful to the researchers and practitioners who will do the work that remains.

12.2 What the Research Taught the Researcher?

The research taught me, first and most persistently, that patients are more interesting than diseases. The burden studies, the caregiver quality of life research, the adherence barrier surveys, the pharmaceutical care outcome measurements: all of them, at their best, were exercises in listening to what patients and caregivers were actually experiencing, which was almost always more complex, more contextually specific and more humanly significant than any clinical metric could fully capture. The dialysis patient managing 12 oral medications and three parenteral medications three times a week at the kidney centre is not a CKD case. She is a person whose treatment has become the dominant structure of her daily life, and whose capacity to sustain that structure depends on social, economic and emotional resources that the clinic's HbA1c target does not address. Research that forgets this is technically competent but humanly inadequate.

The research taught me that institutions matter as much as individuals. A pharmacist with excellent training, genuine commitment to patient-centred practice, and a well-developed pharmaceutical care philosophy will not consistently deliver pharmaceutical care in an environment that does not support, expect or remunerate it. The unit of change in pharmacy practice is not the individual practitioner. It is the system within which the practitioner works: the remuneration structure, the legal framework, the physical environment of the pharmacy, the professional culture and the relationship with other health professionals that either enables or forecloses the kind of patient-centred interaction that pharmaceutical care requires. This insight, confirmed by study after study across the chapters of this book, has direct implications for how research energy should be allocated: more implementation science, more regulatory analysis, more economic modelling of what pharmaceutical care services actually cost and what they save and less self-congratulation about attitudes and knowledge that never reach the patient.

The research taught me that the obligation to patients does not end at publication. A finding that is published and not acted upon has not yet fulfilled its purpose. A protocol that was registered but whose full outcomes have not been published has left an obligation outstanding. A baseline study whose post-implementation comparison has not been conducted has answered half a question. A capacity-building programme whose longitudinal outcomes have not been evaluated has demonstrated education without demonstrating impact. These are not shameful failures; they are the normal incompleteness of research programmes that exist in real institutions, with real constraints on time, funding and follow-through. But naming them honestly, as this book has attempted to do, is the minimum that intellectual accountability requires.

The research taught me, finally, that rigour and reflexivity are not in competition. A researcher can be methodologically rigorous and at the same time honest about the limitations of what their methods can reveal. A research tradition can accumulate a substantial evidence base and at the same time acknowledge that the evidence has not yet produced the practice change it pointed toward. The pharmacy practice research community in the Arab Middle East has, over the period this book documents, built something genuinely valuable: a regional evidence base, a cadre of trained researchers, an institutional infrastructure for producing and publishing health services research. Acknowledging that this achievement has not yet translated into consistent pharmaceutical care practice in the settings where patients need it most is not a denial of the achievement. It is the honesty that the achievement requires, if it is to be more than self-referential.

12.3 The Research Agenda Notes: A Collective Contribution

Each of the 11 substantive chapters in this book closes with a Research Agenda Note containing five open questions. Taken together, these notes comprise approximately 55 research questions that represent, in the author's considered judgement, the most important unfinished work arising from this research programme. They are not a wish list. They are a research agenda grounded in the evidence of what was done, what it found and what it could not resolve. Some of them are intervention trials waiting to be designed. Some are measurement studies waiting to be conducted in settings where the measurement has not yet been done. Some are policy analyses waiting for researchers willing to engage with the regulatory and institutional dimensions of pharmaceutical practice that empirical studies too often leave unexamined. Collectively, they represent a scholarly contribution in their own right: not a catalogue of gaps, but a structured argument about where the field's most important next steps lie.

The deliberate decision to include these questions in a published monograph rather than in grant applications or conference presentations reflects a conviction about the purpose of scholarly publishing. If a research retrospective has any unique contribution to make, it is precisely this: the ability to look across a body of work and identify, with the hindsight that a career's worth of evidence provides, the questions that should have been asked sooner and that must be asked now. Prospective research planning, by its nature, cannot see what a retrospective examination can see. This book has tried to see it clearly and to share what it has seen.

12.4 The Unfinished Agenda

This book has been, throughout, an account of unfinished works. The pharmaceutical care reform in the Arab Middle East is unfinished. The medication-related burden research agenda is unfinished. The connection between what is measured in quality of life studies and what is done in clinical practice is unfinished. The evidence base for pharmacist-led interventions in the Gulf cardiovascular setting is unfinished. The transformation of pharmacy education in the MENA region is unfinished. The counselling gap is still a gap waiting to be closed. The adherence intervention research is unfinished. The caregiver support agenda is unfinished. The tobacco cessation pharmacist role is unfinished. The medicines access equity agenda that COVID-19 made visible is unfinished.

This convergence of incompleteness is not coincidental. It reflects the structural reality described in the Introduction to this book: the gap between what pharmacy promises and what patients receive is not a knowledge gap that more evidence will automatically close. It is a structural gap that requires changes in remuneration frameworks, regulatory environments, professional culture and institutional expectations that are outside the direct control of any individual researcher or even any individual research programme. What research can do, and what this book has attempted to do, is make the gap visible with sufficient precision and honesty that the people and institutions with the authority to address it can no longer reasonably claim that they did not know where the problem was.

12.5 A Final Word

Unfinished work is work that still matters, and work that still matters is work that the next generation of researchers, practitioners and educators has the opportunity, and the obligation, to advance.

This book has been one researcher's attempt to account honestly for what was achieved and what remains. It has not resolved the gaps it documented. No single book could. What it has done is name them precisely, trace them across a research programme and a career and argue that naming them precisely is itself a contribution to closing them. The account is incomplete because the work is incomplete. That, finally, is the most honest thing that can be said about a research career: it is always, necessarily, a work in progress. The question is not whether the work is finished. The question is whether it has been done with sufficient rigour, sufficient honesty and sufficient care for the patients at the centre of it to have made the effort worthwhile. The chapters of this book represent the author's best attempt to answer yes.[1]

References

Dokbua S, Dilokthornsakul P, Chaiyakunapruk N, Saini B, Krass I, Dhippayom T (2018) Effects of an asthma self-management support service provided by community pharmacists: a systematic review and meta-analysis. J Managed Care Spec Pharm 24(11):1184–1196

[1]Publications by the author of this book are marked with an asterisk (*) in references.

El Hajj MS, Kaddoura R, Abu Yousef SEA, Orabi B, Awaisu A, AlYafei S, Shami R, Mahfoud ZR (2023) Effectiveness of a structured pharmacist-delivered intervention for patients post-acute coronary syndromes on all-cause hospitalizations and cardiac-related hospital readmissions: a prospective quasi-experimental study. Int J Clin Pharm 45(3):630–640

Jaam M, Mohamed Ibrahim MI, Kheir N, Hadi MA, Diab MI, Awaisu A (2018) Assessing prevalence of and barriers to medication adherence in patients with uncontrolled diabetes attending primary healthcare clinics in Qatar. Primary Care Diabetes 12(2):116–125*

Kheir N, Emmerton L, Shaw JP (2001) Can pharmacists influence the health-related quality of life of patients with asthma? The New Zealand pharmaceutical care experience. Sultan Qaboos Univ Med J 3(2):70–75*

Kheir N, Ghoneim O, Sandridge AL, Al-Ismail M, Hayder S, Al-Rawi F (2012) Quality of life of caregivers of children with autism in Qatar. Autism 16(3):293–298*

Kheir N, Zaidan M, Younes H, El Hajj M, Wilbur K, Jewesson PJ (2008) Pharmacy education and practice in 13 Middle Eastern countries. Am J Pharm Educ 72(6):133*

Yassen AO, Shlaymoon AS, Ghanim Salem N, Shakir SA (2025) Asthma patient education and counselling in community pharmacies in Kurdistan Region, Erbil, Iraq: a cross-sectional study. Int Pharm Acta 8(1):e7

Zidan A, Awaisu A, Kheir N, Mahfoud Z, Kaddoura R, AlYafei S, El Hajj MS (2016) Impact of a pharmacist-delivered discharge and follow-up intervention for patients with acute coronary syndromes in Qatar: a study protocol for a randomised controlled trial. BMJ Open 6(11):e012141*

FSC
www.fsc.org
MIX
Papier | Fördert
gute Waldnutzung
FSC® C083411

Kolibri 360 GmbH
Ferdinand-Jühlke-Straße 7
99095 Erfurt, Deutschland
produktsicherheit@kolibri360.de